ISBN 978-0-331-14028-6
PIBN 11018544

EXPERIMENTAL AND SURGICAL NOTES UPON THE BACTERIOLOGY OF THE UPPER PORTION OF THE ALIMENTARY CANAL, WITH OBSERVATIONS ON THE ESTABLISHMENT THERE OF AN AMICROBIC STATE AS A PRELIMINARY TO OPERATIVE PROCEDURES ON THE STOMACH AND SMALL INTESTINE

BY.

HARVEY CUSHING, M. D.

AND

LOUIS E. LIVINGOOD, M. D.

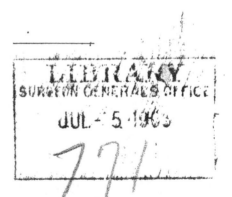

Reprinted from

Contributions to the Science of Medicine, dedicated by his Pupils to William Henry Welch, upon the Twenty-fifth Anniversary of his Doctorate

and

Volume IX of the Johns Hopkins Hospital Reports

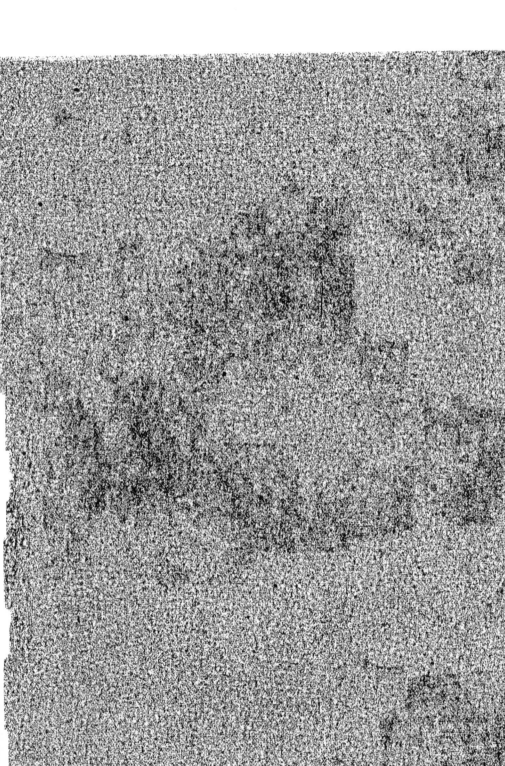

EXPERIMENTAL AND SURGICAL NOTES UPON THE BACTERIOLOGY OF THE UPPER PORTION OF THE ALIMENTARY CANAL, WITH OBSERVATIONS ON THE ESTABLISHMENT THERE OF AN AMICROBIC STATE AS A PRELIMINARY TO OPERATIVE PROCEDURES ON THE STOMACH AND SMALL INTESTINE.

BY

HARVEY CUSHING, M. D.,

Associate in Surgery in the Johns Hopkins University,

AND

LOUIS E. LIVINGOOD, M. D.,

Late Associate in Pathology in the Johns Hopkins University.

Introduction.

In the fall of 1897 there entered the surgical wards of the Johns Hopkins Hospital a young man who had received, *twenty-seven* hours previous to his admission, a gunshot wound in the abdomen. Fortunately, the accident had occurred some hours after the taking of food, and no nourishment had been given since the reception of the injury. Although the patient appeared to be in good condition, and presented no definite symptoms pointing to the existence of any serious intra-abdominal lesion, an exploratory laparotomy disclosed four large intestinal perforations which were all included within the upper few feet of the jejunum. Despite the fact that extravasation of jejunal contents had taken place and that so long an interval had elapsed, there was present but very slight macroscopical evidence of peritonitis, and cultures from the general cavity in the vicinity of the lesions showed merely a few isolated colonies of a staphylococcus. Suture of the perforations and closure of the abdominal parietes without drainage resulted in an uneventful recovery.

The interest aroused by this case led to the tabulation of our complete series of perforating gunshot wounds of the abdomen, which resulted in the surprising demonstration that recovery had followed in those cases alone in which the lesions had been situated at no great distance from the pyloric end of the intestine, whereas all of the cases in our particular series in which the perforations had been far down in the ileum had succumbed to an ensuing peritonitis, though many of them had been operated upon at a comparatively early period and favorable prognoses had been given.

The suggestion derived from these data, that rapidly fatal peritonitides were less likely to follow perforations high up in the canal than similar lesions situated farther down, has led us, since that time, to make routine bacteriological examinations of the contents, especially of the upper portions of the healthy intestine, as opportunities offered themselves at the operating table, with the view of determining, if possible, the nature and pathogenicity of the local bacterial flora and its bearing upon the prognosis of surgical procedures in that portion of the intestine. Experimental observations upon animals were also undertaken with the same object in view, as well as to establish as far as possible the varieties and relative number of micro-organisms in the different parts of the canal at various periods of digestion and the degree to which this flora might be influenced by sterilization of the ingesta and by fasting.

Confession must be made of the feeling of surprise at the discovery (at that time new to the writer at least), that the intestinal canal did not everywhere and at all times contain a host of bacterial forms, pathogenic and otherwise. It was, of course, understood that the particular flora of one portion or another of the tract, depending upon the reaction of digestive secretions, might vary within considerable limits, but the idea that certain areas of the canal might be rendered amicrobic in preparation for operation or might periodically be found so in ordinary conditions of health was novel to us; nor can I find in the literature that the possible importance of these facts has ever been appreciated by abdominal surgeons. Necessarily some extravasation of intestinal contents follows upon perforative lesions of the bowel, whether of traumatic or pathological origin, and also some soiling of the serosa must accompany intentional operative incisions into the lumen. Upon the bacteriological features of this extravasated material depend the nature and degree of the ensuing peritonitis, and consequently the prognosis of the case is favorable in proportion to the scarcity and innocuousness of the micro-organisms which occupy the canal at the level of the lesion.

PERIOD OF AMICROBIC EXISTENCE SUBSEQUENT TO BIRTH AND POSSIBILITY OF ITS CONTINUANCE.

To Billroth[1] is given by Mannaberg[2] the credit of first demonstrating by microscopical studies the sterility of the meconium of new-born babes and the appearance of micro-organisms with the first yellow stools. Not, however, until the fundamental studies of Escherich[3, 4] had established the colon bacillus as the intestinal organism *par excellence*, were any careful cultural observations made upon the bacteriology of the digestive tract. Through his observations, which have since been confirmed by the studies of Schild,[5] Popoff,[6] Szegö[7] and others, it was learned that the intestinal discharges of infants remained sterile after birth for a period of some hours, the duration of which depended apparently upon the interval elapsing before the earliest nourishment was given. Whether the original entry of micro-organisms occurs *per anum* or by the mouth, and if by the latter portal whether through swallowed air, through water taken at the first bath of the infant, or together with its nourishment, has remained a subject of conjecture, and it is noteworthy that none of these investigators have succeeded in determining from the child's surroundings what is the source of supply of B. coli communis, which appears almost among the first bacterial forms in the stools and remains, apparently, the only permanent inhabitant throughout life.

[1] Billroth, Th. Untersuchungen über die Vegetationsformen von Coccobacteria septica u. s. v. Berlin, 1874, S. 94.

[2] Mannaberg. Julius. Die Bakterien des Darms. Nothnagel's specielle Pathologie und Therapie, Bd. XVII, 1 Theil, 1 Abt., S. 17, 1895.

[3] Escherich, Theodor. Die Darmbakterien des Neugeborenen und Säuglings. Fortschritte der Medicin, Bd. III, S. 515 und 547, 1885.

[4] Escherich, Theodor. Die Darmbakterien des Säuglings und ihre Beziehungen zur Physiologie der Verdauung. Stuttgart, 1886.

[5] Schild, Walther. Das Auftreten von Bakterien in Darminhalte Neugeborener vor der ersten Nahrungsaufnahme. Zeitschrift für Hygiene und Infectionskrankheiten, Bd. XIX, S. 113, 1895.

[6] Popoff, D. Die Zeit der Erscheinung und die allmähliche Verbreitung der Mikroorganismen im Verdauungstraktus der Thiere. Wratsch., 1891, No. 39. Centralblatt f. Bakteriologie, Bd. XI, p. 214, 1892.

[7] Szegö, Koloman. Die Darmmikroben der Säuglinge und Kinder. Archiv für Kinderheilkunde, Bd. XXII, S. 25, 1897.

Nuttall and Thierfelder[1] have attempted experimentally to determine whether or not the continuance of the early amicrobic state of the bowel was incompatible with a normal mammalian existence, and though their observations are too few to be conclusive, they nevertheless show that for a time at least an animal may lead an extra-uterine life and be nourished without the presence of bacterial growth in the intestine. For eight days they succeeded in keeping alive and well a guinea-pig which had been obtained by Cæsarean section, confined in a sterile chamber, breathing sterilized air and fed upon sterile milk. At the end of that time the animal was killed and the intestinal contents on microscopical and cultural examination were found to be free from micro-organisms. Such experiments are very difficult to successfully carry out and no confirmation of their results has been forthcoming; in fact, one observer, Schottelius,[2] takes exception to them, as he was unable to maintain life over twenty days in chickens hatched in sterile surroundings. Perhaps the recent communication of Levin[3] may be interpreted as in a manner confirmatory of Nuttall's observations and as upholding the view that intestinal bacteria are unnecessary for the proper assimilation of food, while strongly suggesting that freedom from the ingestion of micro-organisms leads to their absence throughout the digestive tract. Levin studied the intestinal contents of animals in the arctic regions (Spitzbergen); that is, of animals born in surroundings which naturally were almost as amicrobic as were the artificial ones in the case of Nuttall's guinea-pig. The digestive tract of white bears, seals, reindeer, eider-ducks, penguins, etc., were found in most cases entirely sterile. In one white bear and two seals examined, an occasional organism resembling the colon bacillus was found. In the arctic zone the great rarity of micro-organisms in the air and the small number in the water (estimated at 1 organism for 11 cc. of water, while the

[1] Nuttall, Geo. H. F., und H. Thierfelder. Thierisches Leben ohne Bakterien im Verdauungskanal. Zeitschrift für physiologische Chemie. Bd. XXI, S. 109, 1895.

Ibid. II Mittheilungen, Zeitschrift für physiologische Chemie. Vol. XXII, S. 62, 1896.

Ibid. III Mittheilungen. Versuche an Hühnern, Zeitschrift für physiologische Chemie. Vol. XXIII, S. 231, 1897.

[2] Schottelius, Max. Ueber die Bedeutung der Darmbakterien für die Ernährung. Archiv für Hygiene, Bd. XXXIV, S. 210, 1899.

[3] Levin. Les microbes dans les régions arctiques. Annales de l'Institut Pasteur, Tome XIII, p. 558, 25 juillet, 1899.

Seine in contrast has 2,000,000 in the same amount) accounts presumably for the paucity of bacteria ingested and the consequent freedom from an intestinal flora.

First Appearance of Bacteria and the Establishment of an Intestinal Flora.

Under ordinary conditions of animal life, however, as Escherich and later writers have shown, some hours after birth micro-organisms make their appearance in all portions of the digestive tract. Since in healthy individuals of a given species there is a similarity not only in the character of the food, but also in the digestive secretions which act upon it and influence its bacterial elements in various parts of the alimentary canal, it naturally follows that there soon becomes established a recognizable flora which may vary with the species as well as for different portions of the intestinal canal of the individual. Furthermore, as elements constituting this flora, we must recognize two subdivisions, one of which includes the permanent or obligatory intestinal bacteria, and the other, the transient or facultative forms, the former being invariably present, while the latter only appear after being accidentally introduced with the ingesta, and unless they encounter or themselves produce some pathological lesion of the mucosa, do not find in the presence of the permanent flora cultural conditions which favor their perpetuation. The so-called obligatory forms, however, are themselves dependent somewhat upon dietary influences. A familiar illustration is that of human sucklings in whom Escherich showed that B. lactis aërogenes is the obligatory form high up in the canal while B. coli flourishes farther down, all of the other organisms which he isolated apparently being only accidental occupants. This condition, of course, presupposes a diet of the greatest simplicity, and with the change to a more varied food the flora, especially in its transient forms, may become much more irregular. Variations also occur in different species. In many animals—dogs, cats, cows, hogs and others—B. coli and its near allies seem to be, as in man, the chief obligatory forms. For horses, Dyar and Keith[1] have established an especial variety—B. equi intestinalis—which is always present in the dung in great numbers. Again,

[1] Dyar, Harrison G., and Simon C. Keith, Jr. Notes on Normal Intestinal Bacilli of the Horse and of other Domesticated Animals. Technology Quarterly, Vol. VI, No. 3, October, 1893.

in some animals, through dietary peculiarities, transient forms may be few in number or altogether absent from portions of the canal. In rabbits, indeed, it has been a common observation with us to find the upper part of the intestine sterile during active digestion; and Dyar observed that their fæces, as well as those of goats, were not rarely sterile, nor does B. coli, of the accepted type, seem to be a common inhabitant of the ileum, where, however, in these as well as other animals, numerous bacillary forms are ordinarily found.

Lembke[1] has roughly attempted to determine the variations in the intestinal flora of dogs which were fed for a series of days on different foods by comparing the bacterial forms found in the stools after a mixed diet or one of bread, meat, or fat respectively. Considerable differences were found to occur, but his observations are open to the same objection as those of many other investigators, namely, that the varieties of micro-organisms in the fæces can hardly be supposed to represent the flora of those parts of the canal where active digestion goes on. It has been an occasional practice in laboratory teaching at this hospital for the students to make microscopical as well as cultural examinations of their own fæces, and it is astonishing how few of the countless micro-organisms which Nothnagel described, and which seem to make up the chief part of the bulk of the stool, can be cultivated. In agreement are the observations of Bienstock,[2] who was able to isolate only a few bacillary varieties from human fæces. Lembke found, however, that in 81 cases examined, B. coli alone remained constant and independent of diet, though a non-liquefying coccus and a yellow sarcina were seldom missed by him. Though some change could be observed in the relative number of organisms present under a restricted diet, with the return to the usual food the original organisms were found once more to become the predominating ones.

Just why the colon bacillus persists as the peculiar denizen of the lower bowel in most animals is as difficult of explanation as is the source of its early appearance in the infant's intestine. Claudio Fermi[3] and others have offered many hypotheses, none of which

[1] Lembke, W. Beitrag zur Bacterienflora des Darms. Archiv f. Hygiene, Bd. XXVI, S. 293, 1896.

[2] Bienstock. Ueber die Bakterien der Fæces. Zeitschrift für klin. Med., Bd. VII, 1884.

[3] Fermi, Claudio. Ueber die Ursachen, welche die Beständigkeit der Flora intestinalis in Bezug auf die Immunität gegen Cholera feststellen. Centralblatt für Bakteriologie, Bd. XVIII, No. 23, S. 705, 1895.

is entirely satisfactory. It is an organism, however, which retains its viability under very adverse circumstances; it is an acid-producer and can survive in an acid medium destructive to many other bacteria. The vigor of its growth is well shown by the ease with which it overgrows other intestinal organisms when a fair field is supplied, such as the peritoneum offers after an intestinal perforation, as well as in similar conditions *in vitro*, as it will rapidly outstrip most others, with few exceptions, in bouillon inoculated with polymorphous varieties.

Aside from this ever-presiding colon bacillus and possibly one or two of the forms which Macfayden and Ciechomski[1] have found present with some constancy, it does not seem natural to regard other micro-organisms which may be encountered in the intestine as more than accidental forms. One might almost as well regard cultures taken from food and water before ingestion as indicative of the varieties of intestinal bacteria.

Gessner[2] has attempted to establish a definite duodenal flora for man, his observations having been made upon the intestinal contents of cadavers, on many occasions after recent death from trauma. No note, however, is made of the stage of digestion, and many of the organisms described by him are doubtless transient inhabitants and are not to be regarded as essential members of the local flora. Unfortunately no mention is made by Gessner of stained preparations, and the relative number of bacteria consequently is not obtainable. From several post-mortem studies upon recent deaths Dr. Livingood obtained such conflicting results in the duodenal observations that this method of obtaining data was abandoned. On one or two occasions, however, sterile duodenums were encountered accompanying an empty stomach, but when the latter contained liquid nourishment, as was usually the case, the duodenal flora was found to be a most variable one.

Macfayden, Nencki and Sieber[3] accepted the opportunity offered

[1] Ciechomski, A. und M. Jakowski. Ungewöhnlich lange dauernde kunstlicher After, nebst chemisch-bacteriologischen Untersuchung über den Inhalt der Düngdärme. Archiv für klinische Chirurgie, Bd. XLVIII. S. 136, 1894.

[2] Gessner, C. Ueber die Bakterien im Duodenum des Menschen. Archiv für Hygiene. Bd. IX. S. 128, 1889.

[3] Macfayden, A., M. Nencki und Sieber. Untersuchungen über die chemischen Vorgänge im menschlichen Düngdarm. Archiv für experi-

by a case in Kocher's clinic, in which a complete intestinal fistula in the ileocæcal region was present, to investigate the intestinal reactions and bacteriology of the discharge at this situation. They first demonstrated the acid reaction of the intestinal contents at this lowest level of the small bowel and isolated six varieties of bacilli and a liquefying streptococcus. Variations in diet made hardly any appreciable difference in the character of this flora, and an observation under similar conditions made by Ciechomski and Jakowski gave results, chemical and bacteriological, similar to those of Macfayden. In three of the cases to be reported in our series, which presented complete fistulæ, I have not been able to convince myself that there exists a peculiar and stable flora, though exceptional advantages were offered for its determination and the fistulæ were in various situations high up in the tract. In fact, all of the forms present might be considered to be facultative, since it was possible to completely remove all bacteria by establishing a sterile dietary régime, followed by a fast long enough to allow the bowel to empty itself. This, however, will be dwelt upon later. It is noteworthy, also, that the lower limb of the fistula in all cases, necessarily being empty, was found at the operation to be sterile. Had there existed in that situation a stable flora in the ordinary conception of the term, one would have expected to find the customary organisms persisting, especially as here the supposed inhibitory action of the gastric secretions was no longer in operation.

Fermi, Brotzu,[1] Dallemagne,[2] Gessner, Macfayden, Gilbert and Lion,[3] with others, have all similarly tabulated, from one situation or another, organisms supposed to be representative of the local intestinal flora, but, as has been stated, leaving aside the probable persistence of B. coli in the lower part of the canal where some of the intestinal contents presumably always remain, it seems most

mentelle Pathologie und Pharmakologie, Bd. XXVIII, Heft 3 u. 4, S. 311, April 2, 1891. Cf. Journ. of Anat. and Physiol., Vol. XXV.

[1] Brotzu, Luigi. Sulla disinfezione del canale intestinale. Annali dele' instituto d'igiene sperimentale della R. Universita di Roma. Vol. IV (Nuova serie), p. 427, 1894.

[2] Dallemagne, J. Contribution à l'étude des microbes du tube gastro-intestinal des cadavres. Bulletin de l'académie royale de médecine de Belgique. Tome VIII, p. 749, 1894. Also Archives de médecine expérimentale et d'anatomie pathologique, 1895, p. 274.

[3] Gilbert et Lion. Contribution a l'étude des bactéries intestinalis. Mémoires de la Soc. de Biol., 9e serie, T. V, p. 55, 1893.

proper to regard in adult life the presence of all other organisms as resultant to a purely fortuitous introduction with the food.[1]

Relative Number of Micro-organisms in Different Portions of the Canal During Periods of Digestion and Fasting.

We have seen, therefore, that following upon the first introduction of nourishment there becomes established a bacterial flora, the elements of which vary within such wide limits, and which, in certain parts of the canal at all events, are so entirely dependent upon the bacteriology of the ingesta that permanent organisms, if any such exist, are unrecognizable. There remains, however, one definite characteristic, namely, that notwithstanding the number of varieties which may be found at one level or another of the canal, the relative numbers of micro-organisms at different situations retain, during periods or intervals of digestion, a more or less definite proportion.

Cognizance has been taken of this by Marfan and Bernard,[2] by Gilbert and Dominici,[3] and the latter have endeavored to diagrammatically represent, by a curve, the relative number of bacteria which are present in the contents of different parts of the tract. Gilbert's observations were made upon dogs which were killed

[1] It must be remembered that we are considering a normal condition of the alimentary canal. In pathological states a second source of entry must be born in mind, namely, by way of the biliary passages after elimination through the liver of bacteria which are present in the blood. Under these circumstances naturally the direct action of the gastric juice is avoided. Buchner (Beiträge zur Kenntniss der Neapoler Cholerabacillen. Arch. f. Hygiene, Bd. III, 1885) demonstrated, for example, that cholera vibrios, which are very non-resistant to the action of gastric juice, could be recovered from the intestine of guinea-pigs after intravenous inoculation. Similar observations have been made by the writer with B. typhosus and members of the hog cholera group (cf. rabbit IX of the series in this paper and pathological report on animals in The Journal of Experimental Medicine). In conditions of health, however, with which alone we have attempted to deal in this paper, such a portal of entry can be left out of consideration.

[2] Marfan, A.-B. et Léon Bernard. Bactériologie de l'intestin. Absence des microbes dans la muqueuse intestinale normale des animaux. Caractère pathologique de leur présence. La Presse Médicale, 10 mai, 1899, p. 217.

[3] Gilbert et Dominici. Réchérches sur le nombre des microbes du tube digestif. Bull. de la Société de Biologie, 10 février, 1894, p. 117.

three hours after taking a meal of bread and meat. Examination of the intestinal contents at this stage of digestion showed an abundance of organisms in the stomach, a pronounced diminution in number at the duodenum, followed by a gradual increase to the ileocæcal valve, where bacteria flourish in the greatest luxuriance. When the large intestine is reached there is a marked falling off in number, with a slight rise proportionate to the distance from the cæcum.

One feature of this curve, namely, the rapid rise at the ileocæcal region of the small bowel, where invariably in health the microbic life is most abundant, remains the same apparently for

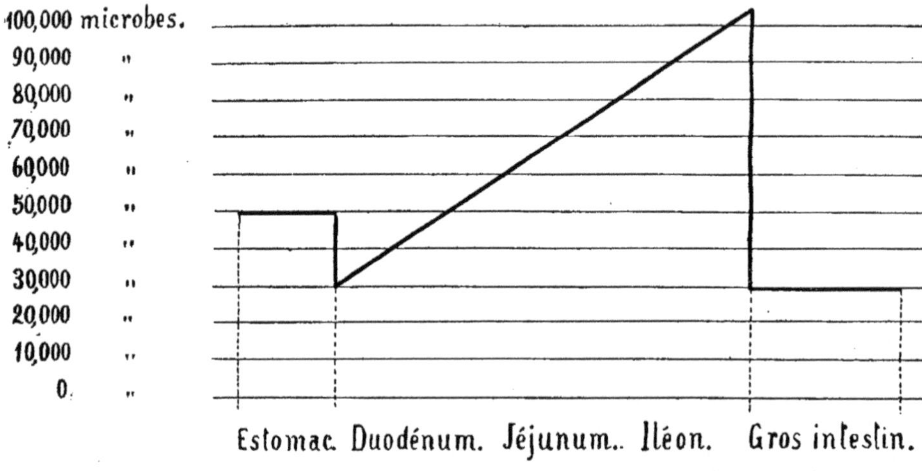

Diagram of Gilbert and Dominici, showing the relative number of micro-organisms in the dog's intestine two or three hours after a meal. (Société de Biologie. Séance du 10 février, 1894.)

all animals and under all conditions except those accompanying disease. The first and last part of the curve may vary greatly with the period of digestion, the flora of the ingesta and the animal species of the host. In rabbits, for example, as Gilbert stated, we find ordinarily a much less abundant flora than in animals living on a more varied diet. It has been our experience to find the duodenum of rabbits amicrobic, even in the active stage of digestion, although the ileum always contained many bacteria. Dyar also found the stools of these animals not infrequently sterile. A diagrammatic representation, therefore, of the number of forms at various levels of the rabbit's canal would often present two amicrobic areas.

Various circumstances tend to bring about this result; the animals used are healthy, kept in clean cages and fed upon fresh vegetables, and doubtless the flora of the ingesta, compared with that of dogs eating ill-cooked mixed diet picked up from floors, would be very scanty. Again, very little liquid food is taken and presumably the material which stays for a long time in the stomach may thus have the full benefit of prolonged antagonism of the gastric juice toward its contained bacteria.

It can be seen by consulting our observations upon dogs that amicrobic areas similar to those ordinarily found in the rabbit may be brought about in other animals by dietary restrictions, so that evidently the character of the curve representing the relative number of bacteria at different levels is a fluctuating one which may vary not only with the species but according to circumstances with the individual. One fact remains certain, however, that the greatest number of bacteria lurk in the lower part of the small intestine and that under all circumstances in health there is a relative scarcity in the duodenum.

Influences Determining the Relative Scarcity of Bacteria in the Upper Portions of the Canal.

I. *Digestive secretions.*—To the digestive secretions naturally one looks for protection against an overwhelming bacterial invasion of the alimentary canal, but it has been found that even in the case of the chief bactericidal factor, the gastric juice, there are many limitations to this protective agency. Although in the stomach during digestion there is undoubtedly a great falling off in the absolute number of micro-organisms, as Miller,[1] Gillespie[2] and others have shown, still even at the height of digestion, two hours after a meal and the stomachs of animals, according to Capitan and Moran,[3] contain a great number of bacteria.

Macfayden's[4] experiments tend to show that the hydrochloric

[1] Miller, W. D. Die Mikroorganismen der Mundhöhle. 2. Aufl. Leipzig, bei Thieme, 1892.

[2] Gillespie. A. Lockhart. The Bacteria of the Stomach. The Journal of Pathology and Bacteriology. Vol. I. p. 279. 1893.

[3] Capitan et Moran. Récherches sur les micro-organismes de l'estomac. Comptes Rendus Hebd. de la Société de Biologie, Séance du 12 janvier. Année. 1889, p. 26.

[4] Macfayden, Allen. The Behavior of Bacteria in the Digestive Tract. Journal of Anatomy and Physiology, Vol. XXI, p. 227, January, 1887.

acid alone is the germicidal factor in producing this diminution in the number of organisms, which progresses, according to Gillespie, proportionately with the increase in total acidity in the gastric juice; furthermore, Miller, after purposely introducing bacteria into the stomachs of animals, was able to demonstrate a progressive decrease in the number of recoverable organisms so that, after the end of nine hours, no return whatever is obtained. Influences other than antisepticity of gastric juice, however, might account for this terminal stage of amicrobism, since Macfayden, Fermi[1] and others have shown that hypho- and blastomyces, as well as many bacteria, often pathogenic ones, as the staphylococci, B. typhosus and others, are resistant to even a greater degree of acidity than that found even in those animals in which it reaches its highest percentage during digestion. Consequently, under most favorable circumstances the bactericidal effect of the gastric juice has marked limitations. When the duodenum is reached, however, as Gilbert's diagram shows, there is, even during the early hours of digestion and when the stomach contains a great multitude of pleomorphic organisms, a distinct falling off in the relative number of bacteria. This relative diminution, Gilbert and Dominici, Escherich and others have believed to be due simply to the dilution of the chyme by the biliary and pancreatic fluids, since the bactericidal action of these secretions contrary to former physiological beliefs, is barely appreciable.[2]

[1] Fermi, Claudio. Die Mineral- und organischen Säuren, die Alkali, die Alkaloide, das Jodkali und das arsensaure Kali zur Differenzierung der Mikroorganismen. Centralblatt für Bakteriologie, Bd. XXIII, Abth. I, S. 208, 1898.

[2] Bile has long been considered by physiologists to play a considerable rôle in combating bacterial growth in the intestine. It has been shown, however, that complete biliary fistulæ may persist without seriously interfering with digestive processes. (Cf., Franz Pfaff and A. W. Balch, Journal of Experimental Medicine, Vol. II, p. 49.) Furthermore, that bile has no inhibitory effect upon many of the more common pathogenic bacteria has been shown *in vitro;* and the fact is well illustrated by the persistence of certain organisms, as B. typhosus and B. coli, in the gall-bladder of infected individuals. Case I of our operative series (to follow), in which a complete common-duct obstruction existed, and in which the duodenum was found as amicrobic as in many other cases in which bile had passed freely into the bowel, would speak against any possible action of the bile in bringing about such a condition. Leubuscher (Einfluss von Verdauungssecreten auf Bakterien. Zeitschrift für klinische Medicin, Bd. XVII, S. 472, 1890) found that yeasts alone grew poorly in the pres-

The influence of this dilution is not far-reaching, but is gradually overcome, as the chyme passes downward, partly by absorption and partly by the renewed multiplication of bacteria which doubtless find less antagonism to growth as the pronounced acidity of the upper portion of the canal is diminished in proportion as the contents approach to the large intestine.

II. *Character of ingesta.*—It would seem, therefore, necessary, since the germicidal action of the secretions has such limitations, that we take into especial consideration in the study of the flora of the upper part of the tract, on the one hand, the physical characteristics of the food, since the length of time during which it remains in the presence of the gastric juice depends largely upon its fluidity, and also the number of bacteria introduced with it. Micro-organisms in liquid medium or taken at the beginning of a meal are rapidly passed, unaffected by the gastric secretions, into the duodenum and intestine where they become, at all events, transient inhabitants, and it is easily seen that a liquid diet would favor the early passage of bacteria through the pylorus.

In one of the cases of jejunal fistula, in our series, it was remarkable to see how rapidly the stomach emptied itself of simple fluid contents. Within a few minutes after its ingestion a glass of milk could be entirely recovered at the fistula, its bacteriological features practically unchanged. Macfayden has shown that anthrax, an organism easily killed by the action of gastric juice, cannot be recovered from the intestine when taken after a full meal, but that, when administered with a large amount of liquid on an empty stomach, its recovery from the lower bowel is readily accomplished. Ewald has, I believe, demonstrated a similar possibility in the case of cholera vibrios. In one of our cases, B. prodigiosus, an organism especially susceptible to the action of the gastric juice, could be easily recovered from a jejunal fistula after its ingestion with inoculated milk. Under such circumstances, therefore, it is readily seen that the flora of the fluid ingesta may entirely escape any bactericidal effect whatever on the part of the gastric secretion, which, even

ence of bile, which may account for the disappearance of these forms from the intestinal flora. Free bile acids, however, he found to possess on the contrary true bactericidal action, so that the old idea of disinfection is in a manner justifiable, provided that conditions are present in the progress of digestion to allow of their liberation.

under most favorable circumstances, when undiluted, is very incomplete in its action.

III. *Period of digestion, especially that of the terminal emptying of the canal.*—It can be readily understood, therefore, that the number of micro-organisms which escape digestive action in the stomach bear an important relation to the stage of digestion. Early in the process, and especially with a liquid diet, a great number and variety of forms may be recovered from the duodenum. Late in digestion, and with a dry diet, we may find that relatively few viable organisms pass the pylorus, the gastric juice under these circumstances having a most favorable opportunity of exercising its germicidal action. Another factor, however, I believe, underlies the terminal condition of amicrobism of the stomach which succeeds, as Miller's experiments demonstrated, the gradual diminution in the number of bacteria during digestion. It is difficult for us to conceive of a glandular surface so thoroughly strewn with micro-organisms as is the gastric and duodenal mucosa during the digestive process, becoming in a comparatively short time practically free from micro-organisms. Marfan and Barnard,[1] however, have recently conducted some researches which throw light upon this subject. Having confirmed previous observations as to the entry of micro-organisms into the intestinal mucosa during pathological processes, these writers undertook experiments which showed that in a state of health the mucous membrane was absolutely amicrobic. Only after artificially induced enteritides (in their cases by arsenic) and in pathological states could micro-organisms be demonstrated occupying the mouths of the mucous glands. Here, then, we have a condition unlike that obtaining in the skin, with its definite glandular flora, since micro-organisms do not lurk in the recesses below the surface of the mucous membranes, and it is easily understood how it becomes possible for a viscus like the stomach to completely free itself of all bacterial life, as the terminal products of digestion are swept along through the pylorus, and how a similar condition of amicrobism of the lumen may be arrived at through the agency of the peristalsis as far down as complete emptying of the canal of products which carry or sustain bacterial life may be brought about. Under ordinary circumstances of life, naturally, since the periods of taking

[1] Marfan et Bernard. La Presse Médicale, 10 mai, 1899, p. 217.

food follow each other at fairly close intervals, and since the buccal flora is periodically swallowed with the saliva, the absolute emptying from food and bacteria even of the stomach only rarely occurs, so that it is unusual for this condition of terminal amicrobism to be arrived at. Exceptionally, however, occasions may arise after periods of enforced fasting in which this resultant amicrobic state may be encountered in the stomach, as is illustrated by the following cases which were especially favorable for the bacteriological examination of a healthy gastric mucosa under the conditions we are discussing:

I. Gastrostomy for peach stone impacted at the cardiac orifice of the stomach. No food for 12 hours.

II. Gastrostomy for impermeable stricture of the œsophagus in an adult. Prolonged fast.

III. Gastrostomy for impermeable recent lye stricture in a child. Nourishment refused for many hours.

IV. Gastrostomy for dilatation of œsophageal stricture in a child. Preliminary fast for 6 hours.

V. Gastrostomy for impermeable traumatic stricture in an adult. No nourishment retained for many hours.

In all these cases, without exception, the small amount of material which could be obtained from the mucous surface of the stomach at the time of operation proved to be amicrobic on microscopical and cultural examinations. There would seem, therefore, to be a tendency on the part of the stomach to completely free itself, together with the end products of digestion, from even those microorganisms which are resistant to the gastric juice, and, consequently, to speak of the natural flora of the stomach is inappropriate, since in its natural empty state in health the viscus becomes amicrobic. Schlatter's, Brigham's and other cases of total extirpation of the stomach show that, irrespective of the action of the gastric juice in keeping down bacterial life, digestive processes may continue to a degree sufficient to maintain health. It is, I believe, dependent only upon interference with the stomach's power to completely expel its contents that bacterial life may persist in its lumen. The same principle holds true for the duodenum, and it is not improbable that a similar amicrobic stage following digestion with a canal completely free from food and the accompanying bacteria may be brought about as far down as a condition of emptiness may be reached through fasting.

Three opportunities have offered themselves in the past year to demonstrate the sterility of the portion of the intestine which constituted the distal loop of a complete fistula. In each case, no food having ever been administered by the lower loop of the bowel, at the time of operation and resection, scrapings from the surface of the mucous membrane at some distance from the fistula proved to be amicrobic. In none of these cases after the establishment of the fistula had the lower limb been utilized for purposes of feeding, and there had been a complete escape of digestive products by the proximal limb. Consequently, at the time of resection and suture, the lower part of the bowel, being in a state of prolonged fasting, was found to be absolutely free from micro-organisms, microscopical and cultural examination of the scrapings from the surface of the mucosa proving negative at the seat of resection several inches from the fistula. These fistulæ were presumably all jejunal, but situated at different levels of the canal, and the evidence that no bacterial life whatever tended to remain on the mucosa and to resist the propulsive action of the bowel would argue against the existence of any natural flora other than that furnished by the ingesta.

Discussion of the Question of Disinfection and a Natural Method of Accomplishing it.

The advocacy of various so-called intestinal antiseptics, too numerous to mention, is difficult to understand in the face of experimental work undertaken in the vain attempt to establish any efficiency whatever toward the sterilization of the alimentary canal by any of those drugs ordinarily employed for this purpose. Sucksdorff,[1] Stern[2] Brotzu, Albu[3] and many others who have undertaken this work have come to the conclusion, from experimental evidence on man and animals, that only by the sterilization of food and consequent diminution in the number of introduced bacteria, could any definite decrease in the number of intestinal micro-organisms be demonstrated.

[1] Sucksdorff, Wilhelm. Das quantitative Vorkommen von Spaltpilzen im menschlichen Darmkanale. Archiv für Hygiene, Bd. IV, S. 355, 1886,

[2] Stern, Richard. Ueber Disinfection des Darmcanales. Zeitschrift für Hygiene und Infectionskrankheiten, Bd. XII, S. 88, 1892.

[3] Albu, Albert. Zur Frage der Disinfection des Darmcanals. Berliner klinische Wochenschrift, Bd. XXXII, No. 44, S. 958, 1895.

Credit is due to pædiatrists for their adoption of more rational principles in the avoidance of, as well as in the treatment of, intestinal disorders in children. Gilbert and Dominici[14] have shown that a simple milk diet, which presumably greatly lessens the varieties of micro-organisms introduced, has a remarkable effect in causing a diminution of the number in the fæces, in both man and animals. In one case, 67,000 bacteria per milligram represented the number in the fæces in ordinary conditions of alimentation; after two days of a simple milk diet the number fell to 14,000, after three to 5,000, four to 4,000, and after five days to 2,250. In a case of ulcer of the stomach in which a sterilized milk diet was administered, the diminution was much more rapid. They believed that a corresponding condition of comparative freedom from bacterial life existed at the same time throughout the intestinal tract, and succeeded in demonstrating it in the case of dogs. On one occasion a dog fed exclusively on milk for a period of two weeks showed a relative falling off in number as follows:

	Mixed diet.	After milk diet.
Stomach	50,000 germs per mg.	100 germs.
Duodenum	30,000 " " "	50 "
Ileum	100,000 " " "	1300 "
Large Intestine	30,000 " " "	1275 "

Similar results have been arrived at by other observers. Sucksdorff, for example, found the number of bacteria in the stools on ordinary diet to vary between 2,300,000, the maximum, and 25,000 the minimum, while after a sterilized diet these numbers fell to 15,000 as the maximum and 53 as the minimum per milligram of fæces. Only questionable results followed upon the administration in his hands of ordinary so-called antiseptics. Confirmatory evidence, therefore, is given of what has been maintained in the foregoing paragraphs, namely, that the number of micro-organisms in the canal depends, in health, largely upon the number introduced by the mouth and not upon the multiplication of the pre-existing bacteria in the medium for growth afforded by the intestinal contents.

Gilbert's diagram and figures, which have been quoted, represent approximately the number of bacteria present at different levels

[1] Gilbert et Dominici. Action du régime lacté sur le microbisme du tube digestif. Bull. de la Société de Biologie, 14 avril, 1894, p. 277.

during active digestion, and also illustrate the absolute decrease in numbers occurring under dietary restrictions. The following observation was made with a view of determining the nature of the curve representing the relative number of bacteria some hours after the cessation of the digestive process.

Observation upon the Number of Organisms in a Dog's Intestine after a 24 Hours' Fast.

February 13, 1899. A large, healthy dog, previously fed upon a milk diet, was kept without food for 24 hours, prepared for operation and anæsthetized. The following procedures were then carried out. The canal was opened successively in eleven places from stomach to rectum, and as nearly as possible equal amounts of the contents at the different sites were inoculated into agar tubes, from which aërobic and anaërobic plates were immediately made. An ordinary platinum loop full of material was taken from each situation, and, at the same time, two preparations were made for microscopical examination. Observations were thus made from the stomach, from the duodenum 5 cm. below the pylorus, from the jejunum and ileum, 50 cm., 100 cm., 150 cm., 240 cm. and 330 cm. respectively, below the duodenum, as well as from the lowest part of the ileum 10 cm. above the cæcum, from the ascending colon and rectum. Presection sutures were placed in the bowel in each instance before making the incisions and taking the cultures. The openings were thus immediately closed, as was subsequently the abdominal wall. The following results, microscopical and cultural, were obtained with the assistance of Dr. Clopton. (See table on opposite page.)

These results are represented diagrammatically by the accompanying figure, page 562, which may be compared with that on page 552.

The animal died five days subsequent to the operation. At autopsy the diffuse purulent peritonitis, which was present, had apparently originated from the cæcal suture, since this one alone was found to have broken down. All the other sutures were intact and the most advanced degree of peritonitis was present in the right iliac region. The cultural flora from the general cavity was indistinguishable from that previously found in the lumen of the cæcum.

Although representing but a single observation, this experiment satisfactorily illustrates many of the points dwelt upon heretofore with respect to the comparative freedom of the upper part of the

Situation.	Stained preparation.	Culture.	Organisms.
1. *Stomach.*	Occasional coccus; one faintly staining bacillus.	Sterile.	....
2. *Duodenum.*	Doubtful diplococcus; occasional yeast granule.	8 colonies.	Seven yeast (orange), one sarcina.
3. *Jejunum.* 50 cm. below (2).	Few diplococci; do not decol. by Gram.	3 colonies.	Two yeast; 1 colony of a liquefying bacillus, probably B. subtilis contamination.
4 *Jejunum.* 100 cm. below (2).	Only an occasional yeast granule seen.	174 colonies.	Apparently all yeast.
5. *Jejunum.* 150 cm. below (2).	Occasional doubtful diplococcus.	Sterile.	....
6. *Ileum.* 240 cm. below (2).	Occasional bacillus and yeast granules. Not decolorized by Gram.	63 colonies, two varieties.	Medium-sized unidentified bacillus. No growth from 2nd variety of bacilli.
7. *Ileum* 330 cm. below (2).	Large bacillus which stains by Gram; also an occas. diplococcus; small bacilli of B. coli type.	825 colonies.	Bacilli chiefly unidentified. Allied culturally to B. typhosus.
8. *Ileum.* 10 cm. above val.	Large bacilli and occasional diplococcus which stain by Gram. Diplobacilli.	5,000 colonies, two varieties chiefly.	Bacilli of B. coli type. Unidentified bacillus.
9. *Cœcum.*	Great number of bacteria; pleomorph. bacilli, many staining by Gram. Diplococci; many bacilli of colon type decolorize.	Great number of colonies—100,000 or more.	Plate not worked out. Many liquefy'g bacilli.
10. *Rectum.*	Same morphology as in 9, but fewer in number.	750 colonies.	Not worked out.

canal from micro-organisms; and shows that, even in those animals which ordinarily present an abundant and variable intestinal flora, a portion of the digestive tract may, by a period of fasting, which

40

allows it to become emptied of the products of digestion, become practically amicrobic. It was of no little interest also to find that the subsequent peritoneal infection had originated apparently from the point where the greatest number of bacteria had been encountered at the operation.

Results of Experimental Observations upon Animals.

Owing to the suggestion which was offered by the case mentioned in introducing this paper, a series of observations was instituted in

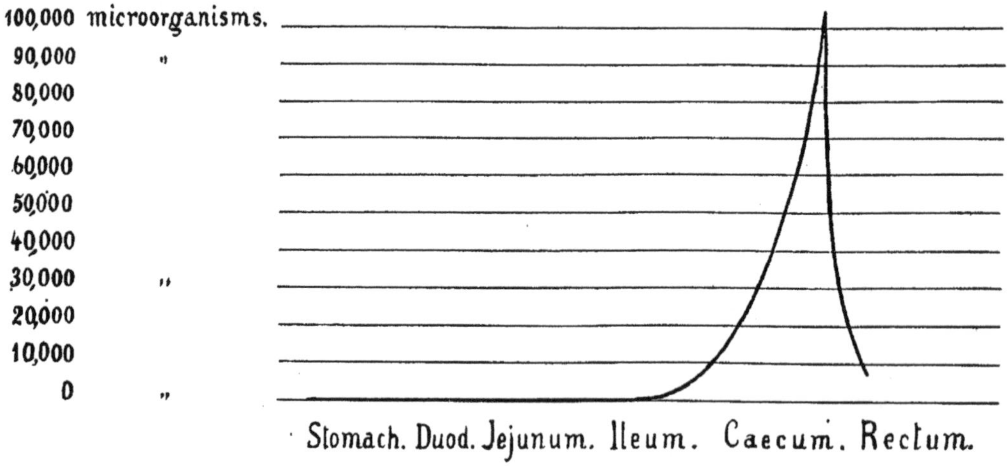

Diagram showing the relative number of micro-organisms at different levels of a dog's intestine after a prolonged fast.

conjunction with Dr. Livingood[1] in the attempt to obtain some data from the investigation of animals relative to the characteristics of the intestinal flora, concerning which we had absolutely no preconceived notions. We decided to limit ourselves chiefly to a comparative study of the number of micro-organisms in the upper and lower portions of the small intestine and to observations upon the

[1] These experiments were carried on during the spring of 1898, with the assistance of Mr. Healy and Mr. Allen of the Medical School, shortly before Dr. Livingood's sad death in the Bourgogne disaster. The large amount of work involved in making such elaborate bacteriological notes as were accumulated could only have been accomplished through the energy and enthusiasm of him whose loss to friends and medicine is irreparable.

nature and pathogenicity of the flora, especially at the former region. For this purpose we examined bacteriologically the intestinal contents of numerous animals at a definite part of the duodenum, eight centimetres below the pylorus, and of the ileum at a similar distance above the cæcum. Synopses of our results are given in the accompanying tables. Unless otherwise specified in the first syllabus, the observations were made upon animals which were laparotomized without any preliminary intestinal preparation, and consequently all stages of the digestive process were encountered. Notes, however, were invariably made upon the probable state of digestive activity as evidenced by the gastric contents, by the amount of material in the duodenum and by the injection of the lacteals; subsequently, observations were made upon animals after intentional dietary restrictions. In the majority of instances the following procedures were carried out: After a hypodermic injection of morphia, the animal was anæsthetized; the abdomen was then prepared for operation, opened and cultures were made through small incisions at the two sites mentioned. In order to establish a certain degree of uniformity in the amount of material taken for cultural purposes, a platinum loop with a diameter of two millimetres was used and the material which its circle would gather up taken as a standard. With this material two melted agar tubes for aërobic and anaërobic growth were inoculated and immediately plated. Two smear preparations for microscopic examination were also made, one for Gram's stain. In this way alone, by examination of stained preparations as a control for the number of colonies on the plates, could any clear conception be formed as to the actual number of organisms present. Frequently bacteria found on the stained preparation afforded no cultural growth, and, indeed, the duodenal flora proved to be so scanty, even in conditions of active digestion, that upon some occasions we allowed the organisms to grow out in bouillon for a few hours before plating them, in order to more surely obtain the prevailing forms. In this way we may have recovered certain bacteria which would have been lost on agar plates.

Several points touched upon in the foregoing pages are illustrated in one way or another by the 35 observations summarized in these first two tables. (1) The comparative scarcity of micro-organisms in the upper part of the canal in both species of animals, even under

TABLE I.

OBSERVATIONS UPON 27 DOGS—TO SHOW THE COMPARATIVE NUMBER AND VARIETY OF BACTERIA OF DUODENUM AND ILEUM.

Nos. and conditions of observation.	Duodenum.		Ileum.		Remarks.
	Microscopical examination.	Number and variety of colonies on plates.	Microscopical examination.	Number and variety of colonies on plates.	
1. Dog I. Feb. 28, '98. Small bull bitch, previously laminectomized; laparotomy; stomach empty; no dietary precautions.	No organisms found.	Sterile { anaërobic. aërobic.	Compar. few organisms. Bacilli decol. by Gram's.	Great number of colonies, pleomorphic, not worked out.	Died of peritonitis originating at lower suture. *B. coli comm.* isolated from duodenum and peritoneal [cav.
2. Dog II. Mar. 4, '98. Autopsy. Death following prolonged physiological experiment.	Few organisms; bacilli; no cocci found.	Anaërob. plate; 75 colonies. *Staphylococcus* and *B. coli comm.*	Numbers of pleomorphic bacilli; large variety with spores.	Aërobic plate, 75 colonies. *B. typhosus* (*var.*). *Diplococcus* (*var.*).	
3. Dog III. do.	Few organisms found; cocci.	Many colonies. *Staphylococci.*	do.	Myriads of colonies. *B. coli comm.*, etc.	
4. Dog IV. do.	No organisms found.	Sterile { anaërobic. aërobic.	do.	Numerous colonies not worked out.	
5. Dog V. do.	Few organisms. Bacilli and occas. coccus.	Anaërobic plate } Aërobic plate } 100 cols. *B. coli comm.* *B. coli comm.* (*var.*)	Great numbers of pleomorphic organisms.	Many hundred colonies. *B. coli comm.*	
6. Dog VI. Mar. 16, '98. Large white bull bitch; stomach full; active digestion; no dietary precautions; laparotomy; cultures; common duct ligated.	No organisms found. Few questionable diplococci.	Sterile.	Many organisms. Bacilli.	600-700 colonies; not worked out.	
7. Dog VI. Mar. 18, '98. Second laparotomy.	No organisms found.	Sterile.	No observation.		Died of peritonitis, cholecystitis, etc. No bacteriological observation.

Nos. and conditions of observation.	Microscopical examination.	Number and variety of colonies on plates.	Microscopical examination.	Number and variety of colonies on plates.	Remarks.
9. Dog VII. Mar. 23, '98. Same animal; actively digesting; no dietary precautions.	Considerable number of bacillary forms, streptothrices, etc.	Aërobic plate, 175 colonies. *B. coli comm.* (*var.*).	Many bacilli of colon type.	Many colonies. *B. coli comm.* (*var.*).	Many omental adhesions about ileum as result of Operation I. Bile sterile; gall-bladder inoc. with *B. typh.*
10. Dog VII. Mar. 31, '98. Same animal. Inoc. Mar. 23 with typhoid. Six hours after large meal. Animal well; no dietary precautions.	Very few organisms found, occas. diplococcus; 2 medium bacilli.	Plates from 14-hour bouillon. *B. typhosus.*	Great numbers of pleomorphic bacilli.	Plates from 14-hr. bouillon. *B. coli comm.* (*var.*). *B. typhosus.*	Typhoidal cholecystitis; *B. typhosus* in bile in great numbers.
11. Dog XII. Mar. 25, '98. Large mongrel dog. No food for 24 hours; stomach empty; gall-bladder inoculated with *B. typhosus.*	Very few organisms found; small diplococci; 1 streptococcus chain; few large bacilli.	Plate from 24-hour bouillon. Contam. *B. subtilis.*	Great numbers of bacill, spore-bearing, etc.	Plates from 24-hr. bouillon. *B. Proteus.*	Subsequent intestinal resection, cf. Dog XXII.
12. Dog XIV. Mar. 31, '98. Newfoundland pup, on boiled-milk diet; fed 2½ hours before operation; lacteals injected.	Very few organisms; small diplococcus: occasional small bacil: yeast.	Plate from 15-hour old bouillon. *Intermediate bacillus*, (hog cholera type).	Many bacillary forms; abundance of organisms.	Plates from 15-hr. bouillon. *B. coli comm.*	Cf. Dog XXVII.
13. Dog XVII. Apr. 10, '98. Small black and tan. No dietary precautions; stomach full; active digestion.	No organisms found; possible coccus.	Plate direct from duodenum. 20 colonies. *Staphylococcus* (*var.*).	Numerous bacilli of colon type.	Plate from 14-hr. bouillon. *B. coli comm.* (*var.*). *B. proteus.*	
14. Dog XVIII. June 10, '98. Pancreatic operation (Flexner). Duodenotomy; injection of pancreatic duct; no dietary precautions.	Occasional diplococcus. (Flexner.)	Agar slant direct. Motile leptothryx.	No observation.	....	
15. Dog XIX. May 28, '98. Pancreatic operation (Flexner). No dietary precautions. Same as 14.	No organisms found. (Flexner.)	Agar slant direct. Inocula'd with several loops; 15 colonies, *Lactis aërogenes.*	No observation.	.	Killed, June 14. No peritonitis; no adhesions.

TABLE I.—*Continued.*

OBSERVATIONS UPON 27 DOGS—TO SHOW THE COMPARATIVE NUMBER AND VARIETY OF BACTERIA OF I

Nos. and conditions of observation.	Duodenum.		Ileum.	
	Microscopical examination.	Number and variety of colonies on plate.	Microscopical examination.	Number and va of colonies on p
16. Dog XX. June 10, '98. Same as 14.	No organisms found. (Flexner.)	Agar slant direct. Several loops; *Staphylococcus*. Few colonies.	No observation.	....
17. Dog XXI. June 16, '98. Small black dog. No food for 24 hours; stomach empty. Pancreatic opera'n (Flexner).	No organisms identified.	Plate from 24-hour bouillon; yeast. *Streptococci*.	No observation.	....
18. Dog XXII. June 16, '98. Small shaggy black dog. Pancreatic operation (Flexner). No dietary precautions; actively digesting.	Comparatively few organisms. Occas. coccus and bacillus of *B. coli* type.	Plate from 24-hour bouillon. *Staphylococcus*. *B. coli comm.* (*var.*)	No observation.	.
19. Dog XXIII. June 17, '98. Small yellow dog. Pancreatic operation (Flexner). No dietary precautions; stomach empty.	Few organisms; occas. large bacillus. Few doubtful cocci.	Agar slant direct. 2 colonies; *B. coli* (*var.*) Plate from 24-hour bouillon. *Staphylococcus*, *B. coli* (*var.*)	No observation.	
20. Dog XXV. June 20, '98. Small black dog. Previous intestinal resection (6 weeks); fed for 36 hours on boiled milk. Pancreatic operation (Flexner).	Very few organisms; occas. coccus; bacilli of colon type.	Anaërobic plate: 10 colonies *B. typhosus* (*var*). Aërobic plate: 40 colonies *B. typhosus*, *B. typhosus* (*var.*), *B. coli comm.* (*var.*)	No observation.	.
21. Dog XXVI. June 20, '98. Same animal as XII. Condition as in observation 20.	Very few organisms; occas. coccus(?) one large bacillus.	Anaërobic plate sterile. Aërobic plate, 16 colonies *B. coli* (*var.*)	No observation.	.

TABLE I.—*Continued.*

OBSERVATIONS UPON 27 DOGS—TO SHOW THE COMPARATIVE NUMBER AND VARIETY OF BACTERIA OF DUODENUM AND ILEUM.

Nos. and conditions of observation.	Duodenum.		Ileum.		Remarks.
	Microscopical examination.	Number and variety of colonies on plates.	Microscopical examination.	Number and variety of colonies on plates.	
22. Dog XXVII. June 20, '98. Same as XIV. Condition as in observation 20.	Very few organisms; occas. coccus and bacillus. Not decol. by Gram.	Anaërobic plate, 10 colonies; *staphylococcus* (*duod.*) Aërobic plate, 8 colonies; *staphylococcus albus* (*var.*).	No observation.	....	Autopsy June 23, '98. Hemorrhagic pancreatitis; peritonitis. *Streptococcus; B. coli comm.*
23. Dog XXVIII. June 22, '98. Medium sized yellow dog. No dietary precautions; actively digesting. Pancreatic operation (Flexner).	Many large bacillary. forms; cocci, yeast. None decolorized by Gram.	Aërobic plate, 300 colonies; yeast; *staphylococcus; B. coli comm.*	No observation.		Autopsy June 24, '98. Hemorrhagic pancreatitis, etc. Peritonitis, yeast and *streptococcus.*
24. Dog XXX. June 24, '98. Large black and white bitch. No food for 24 hours; stomach empty. Pancreatic operation (Flexner).	No organisms found. Large yeast granules; not decol. by Gram.	Aërobic plate, 2 colonies; yeast. Anaërobic 6 colonies; yeast. *Intermediate bacillus; B. coli* (*var.*).	No observation.		
25. Dog XXXI. June 24, '98. Small black dog. No dietary precautions; stomach empty. Pancreatic operation (Flexner).	No organisms found. Yeast granules.	Anaërobic plate sterile. Aërobic plate, 2 colonies; yeast.	No observation.		June 28, autopsy. Duodenal perforation; gangren. pancreatitis. Bact. of peritoneal cavity polymorphous.
26. Dog XXXII. June 25, '98. Large white dog. No food 24 hours; intestinal resection; cultures from jejunum.	Comparatively few organisms; occas. *coccus;* occas. *streptococcus;* yeast.	Aërobic plate, 7 colonies. Aërobic plate, 5 colonies; yeast; *streptococci.*	No observation.	....	
27. Dog XXXIII. Feb. 13, '99. Black and white setter. Animal without food for 24 hours.	No organisms found.	Aërobic plate, 8 colonies; 7 *yeast;* 1 *sarcina.*	Many polymorphic bacilli. Few cocci.	5,000 colonies *B. coli;* unidentified bacillus.	Stomach empty: sterile; upper few feet of jejunum sterile.

TABLE II.—CORRESPONDING OBSERVATIONS UPON RABBITS.

Nos. and conditions of observation.	Duodenum. Microscopical examination.	Duodenum. Number of colonies upon plate and variety.	Ileum. Microscopical examination.	Ileum. Number of colonies upon plates and variety.	Remarks.
1. Rabbit VIII. Mar. 17, '98, inoc. in ear vein with *B. typh.* Apr. 1, reinoc. with *B. typh.* Apr. 21, Widal positive; laparotomy.	No organisms identified; possible coccus(?)	Agar plate sterile.	Many bacillary forms.	Agar plate negative; no organisms grow in ordinary media.	Bile; sterile; cultures from gall-bladder; evidences of cystitis; clumps of dead organisms.
2. Rabbit IX. Mar. 17, '98, intravenous inoc. with *B. typh.* Mar. 19, laparotomy,	No organisms found.	Aërobic plate sterile; anaërobic plate sterile.	No observation.	..	No organisms found; plates remain sterile.
3. Rabbit IX. Apr. 1, reinoc. with *B. typh.* Laparotomy, June 13.	No organisms identified.	Plates from 18-hour bouillon inoc. with several loops from bowel. *B. typhosus.*	Few bacillary forms, colon type.	Plates from 18-hour bouillon inoc. with one loop from bowel. *B. coli comm.* (*var.*)	*B. typh.* obtained from gall-bladder. Gall-stones.
4. Rabbit X. Mar. 18, '98, laparotomy; actively digesting; cultures; common duct ligated.	Very few organisms; occas. small diplococcus; one or two colon-like bacilli.	Aërobic, anaërobic plates, and bouillon culture are sterile.	Great numbers of pleomorphic organisms, chiefly bacilli; spore forms.	Great numbers of colonies; not worked out.	Died of acute cholecystitis, etc.
5. Rabbit XI. Mar. 22, '98, no dietary precautions.	No organisms found.	Aërobic, anaërobic plates, and bouillon culture are sterile.	Great numbers of bacillary forms, diplococci, etc.	Many colonies; not worked out.	
6. Rabbit XIII. Mar. 26, '98, stomach empty; no food for 24 hours; common duct [ligated.	Two small diplococci and one bacillus found in two fields.	Plates and bouillon culture are sterile.	Great abundance of bacillary forms, chiefly colon type.	Great numbers of colonies.	
7. Rabbit XIII. Mar. 29, dead; stomach full; all-bladder	Many bacillary forms with spores; do not de-	Plate sterile; bouillon contains yeast.	No observation.	....	Bile sterile; peri-

diverse conditions of diet and periods of digestion, will be readily appreciated, especially by reference to the results of the microscopical examinations of the stained preparations taken directly from the bowel. Frequently it was impossible to discover any bacteria whatever on coverslip preparations from the duodenum and but few colonies would appear on the plates. (2) We failed to demonstrate any varieties which might be regarded as representative of a local flora in either situation: in fact, most of the varieties found appeared to be accidental and are, presumably, dependent entirely upon the flora of the ingesta.[1] (3) With an empty duodenum, during a period of fasting, practically no persisting bacterial elements could be demonstrated. During periods of active digestion, on the other hand, in the first series, micro-organisms were often present in considerable numbers, and it was not uncommon under such circumstances to isolate from the ileum as the forms predominating there, the same varieties which the duodenum had furnished. Apparently, therefore, a close though temporary relationship exists between the flora of the ingesta and that of the entire digestive tract. (4) Yeasts and coccal forms of bacteria apparently were least affected by the antiseptic action of the gastric secretions and were the most common varieties found in the duodenum. No marked differences between the colonies upon aërobic and anaërobic plates could be made out. (5) Variations in species due to differences in diet were apparent. In rabbits almost always, in dogs not infrequently, the duodenum was found to be amicrobic. In the latter animals, however, a period of fasting would, with some degree of certainty, establish this condition. (6) Apparently, therefore, micro-organisms do not lurk in or upon the mucous surfaces of an empty canal. (7) Rabbit IX and Dog VII illustrate the possibility of the entry in pathological states through the biliary passages of micro-organisms which are naturally, therefore, but little affected by the gastric juice.

The conclusions which may be drawn as regards the probability of ensuing peritonitides are rather limited in these cases. Most of the animals recovered, and many were subsequently laparotomized for other purposes. It was a common experience on such occasions

[1] Mannaberg says (loc. cit., p. 20) in this connection relative to Sucksdorff's work—"dass im Darm keine autocthone Bakterienvegetation besteht, sondern dass diese wesentlich an die Nahrung gebunden ist und in ihrem Mengenverhältniss von derselben abhängt."

to find that, whereas the upper suture was free, the lower suture in the ileum was surrounded by protective omental adhesions, giving evidence of a more marked reaction at that situation. The animals upon which the pancreatic operations had been performed usually succumbed to peritonitis, from a gangrenous pancreatitis or a broken-down suture. Unfortunately, in these latter cases most of the animals had been allowed liquid nourishment after the operations, and consequently fluctuations in the local flora had occurred so that no distinct relationship could be drawn between the bacteriology of the general cavity and the original local duodenal flora.

In Table III have been gathered the varieties of bacilli which were isolated either from the duodenum, ileum or peritoneal cavity of these animals. Only the results of cultivation upon the various media ordinarily employed for differentiation can be given, though it is well understood that more subtle means are required for the actual identification of many of the allied forms of colon, typhoid and the large intermediate group of bacilli which may be recovered from the intestinal canal. Only an approximate nomenclature, therefore, can be given. One needs only to consult the lists of Gilbert and Lion, Tavel and Lanz,[1] Theobald Smith,[2] Germano and Maurea[3] to appreciate the difficulties in the way of establishing relationship in the colon group alone. Doubtless many organisms failed to grow; one large bacillus quite commonly found both in the duodenum and ileum could never be cultivated, nor could the long fine bacilli often seen low down in the bowel be recovered. In the comparatively few cases in which the colonies from the ileum were worked out, B. coli was obtained ten times. It doubtless was invariably present in the dog's intestine at this situation and apparently in its typical form, though the particular specimens obtained possessed more active motility than is usually seen. Lembke[4,5]

[1] Tavel, E., und Otto Lanz. Ueber die Aetiologic der Peritonitis. Basel und Leipzig, 1893.

[2] Smith, Theobald. Notes on the Bacillus Coli Communis and Related Forms. American Journal of Medical Sciences, September, 1895.

[3] Germano and Maurea. Vergleichende Untersuchungen über den Typhusbacillus und ähnliche Bakterien. Zeigler's Beiträge, Bd. XII, S. 495, 1893.

[4] Lembke, W. Bacterium coli anindolicum und Bacterium coli anaërogenes. Archiv f. Hygiene, Bd. XXVII, S. 384, 1896.

[5] Lembke, W. Weiterer Beitrag zur Bacterienflora des Darms. Archiv f. Hygiene Bd. XXIX, S. 304, 1897.

SOURCE.	Short.	Medium.	Long.	Active.	Sluggish.	None.	Gram's decol.	Marked.	Slight.	Alkalinized.	Rapid.	Slow.	None.	Abundant.	Slight.	Negative	Marked.	Slight.	Negative.	Mkd. No pell.	Mkd. Pellicle.	Slight.	Liquefaction	No liquefac.	Abundant, spreading.	Slight, not spreading.	Invisible.	VARIETIES.
1. Autopsy Duod., Dog I....		+			+		+	+			+				+			+				+		+		+		B. coli communis, diplococcus form.
2. Peritonitis, Dog I........	+			+			+	+			+			+				+			+			+		+		B. coli comm.
3. Op. Duodenum, Dog II....	+			+			+	+				+			+			+			+			+	+			B. coli comm.
4. Op. Ileum, "	+			+			+		+				+			+			+		+			+		+		B. typhosus (var.).
5. Autopsy Ileum, Dog III...	+			+			+	+			+			+				+						+		+		B. coli comm.
6. Op. Duodenum, Dog V (1).	+				+		+	+			+			+				+			+			+		+		B. coli comm.
7. " " " (2).		+			+		+		+				+	+				+				+		+	+			B. coli (var.), not coag. milk.
8. Op. Ileum, Dog V........	+				+		+	+			+			+				+			+			+		+		B. coli comm.
9. Op. Duod., Dog VII, No. 9	+			+			+		+				+	+			+				+			+	+			B. coli (var.), not coag. milk.
10. Op. Ileum, Dog VII, No. 9	+			+			+		+				+	+			+				+			+	+			B. coli (var.) " "
11. Op. Duod., Dog VII, No. 10		+		+			+		+				+									+		+		+		B. typh. (var.), growth on potato.
12. Op. Ileum, Dog VII, No. 10		+				+	+		+		+			+				+		+				+	+			B. coli comm.
13. " " "		+		+			+		+				+									+		+		+		B. typh. (var.), growth on potato.
14. Op. Ileum, Dog XII	+				+		+				+				+			+			+					+		B. proteus.
15. Op. Duodenum, Dog XIV..	+			+			+			+			+	+				+				+		+		+		Intermediate bac., Hog Cholera group.
16. Op. Ileum, Dog XIV......	+				+		+	+			+				+			+			+			+		+		B. coli comm.
17. Op. " Dog XVII	+					+	+	+				+			+			+			+			+	+			B. coli (var.), not coag. milk.
18. Op. Duodenum, Dog XVII.			+		+		+	Unchanged.								+	+			+						+		Leptothrix.
19. Op. " Dog XIX..			+			+	+	+			+			+					+		+			+	+			B. lactis aërogenes.
20. Op. " Dog XXII.	+			+			+		+				+	+				+				+		+			+	B. coli (var.), not coag. milk.
21. Op. " Dog XXIII	+				+		+			+			+	+				+			+			+		+		Intermediate bac., Hog Chol. group.
22. Peritonitis, Dog XXIII....	+			+			+			+			+	+					+		+			+		+		" " "
23. Op. Duodenum, Dog XXV..		+		+			+		+				+			+		+				+		+			+	B. typhosus (var.).
24. " " ..			+	+			+		+				+			+			+			+		+			+	B. typhosus (var.), decol. milk.
25. " " ..		+			+		+	+				+				+	+				+			+	+			Unclassified bacillus.
26. Op. Duodenum, Dog XXVI.	+			+			+	+					+	+			+			+				+			+	" "
27. Peritonitis, Dog XXVII ...		+			+		+	+			+			+			+				+			+	+			B. coli comm.
28. Op. Duodenum, Dog XXVIII	+			+			+	+			+			+				+		+				+	+			B. coli comm.
29. Op. " Dog XXX..		+		+			+			+			+			+		+				+		+			+	B. typhosus (var.) produces indol.
30. Op. " " ..	+			+			+		+				+	+			+				+			+	+			B. coli (var.), not coag. milk.
31. Op. Jejunum, Dog XXXIII			+			+	?			+			+			+				+		+					+	Unclassified bacillus.
32. Ileum, Dog XXXIII.......			+			+	+	+			+			+						+				+	+			B. [illegible].
33. Ileum, Rab. XIII.........			+				—	Unchanged.								+			+			+					+	Unidentified sporogenic bacillus.
34. " "			+				—			"						+			+		+				+			" " "
35. Ileum, Rab. XV......		+				+	+		+				+	+				+			+			+	+			B. coli (var.), not coag. milk.

lays special stress upon two varieties which in dogs' fæces he found with considerable regularity and which he called B. coli anindolicum and B. coli anaërogenes, from the absence of characteristics ordinarily passed by B. coli comm. It is possible that the varieties which we supposed were more closely allied to typhoid and called B. typhosus (var.) may represent these organisms of Lembke.

The comparative frequency, as shown in Table IV, with which varieties of cocci were found in duodenal cultures, tends to confirm the view that these organisms are less seriously antagonized by the gastric juice than are the bacillary forms. Inasmuch as the former organisms are regarded with more dread than the latter because provocative of more virulent peritonitides, the importance of eliminating from the ingesta, by sterilization, cocci which thus readily enter the duodenum, and especially the strepto-variety,[1] as a preliminary preparation for high intestinal operations, is readily understood.

One special small diplococcus form which we agreed to call diplococcus duodenalis, was found almost invariably, though in very small numbers, on coverslips from the dog's duodenum. We were not, however, able on any occasion to cultivate this organism.

A staphylococcus which occasionally appeared in short chains of three or four elements, but which we hesitated to call a streptococcus, was most commonly encountered. This did not prove pathogenic for mice. Staphylococcus pyogenes aureus was never found, though this organism readily passes through the stomach, as was demonstrated in our fistula cases. It probably is an unusual accompaniment of food-products in animals.

Observations upon Surgical Cases Illustrating the Foregoing Principles and Their Adaptation to Intestinal Surgery.

The remainder of this paper will be devoted to brief clinical reports of some of the cases in which opportunities have been offered at the operating-table to make observations relative to the bacteriological questions reviewed above.

[1] The great frequency with which streptococci may be found in such a universal food product as milk has been reported by Eastes (Brit. Med. Journ., Nov. 11, 1899, p. 1341). In 186 specimens obtained from various sources he found these organisms present in 75.2 per cent.

TABLE IV.—TABULATION OF COCCI.

Animal, situation of culture and variety of coccus.			Color by Gram.	Milk.			Gas production.	Indol.	Bouillon.		Gelatin, liquefaction.	Growth on potato.	Remarks.
				Acidity.	Decolorized.	Coagulated.			Turbidity.	Pellicle.			
1. Dog II.	Duodenum.	Staphylococcus.	+	Slight.	Slight.	—	—	—	Slight.	—	—	Invisible.	Not pathogenic for mice.
2. Dog III.	"	Staphylococcus.	+	Slight.	Lower half.	—	—	—	Slight.	—	—	Invisible.	Not pathogenic for mice.
3. Dog VII.	"	Streptococcus (?)	+	Slight.	Lower half.	—	—	—	Slight.	—	—	Invisible.	Not pathogenic for mice.
4. Dog VII.	Ileum.	Streptococcus (?)	+	Slight.	Lower half.	—	—	—	Slight.	—	—	Invisible.	Not pathogenic for mice.
5. Dog XVII.	Duodenum.	Sta hylococcus.	+	Slight.	+	—	—	—	—	—	—	Invisible.	
6. Dog XX.	"	Sta hplococcus.	+	Slight.	Lower third.	—	—	—	Very slight.	—	—	Visible slight.	
7. Dog XXI.	"	Streptococcus.	+	—	—	—	—	—	Considerable.	—	—	Invisible.	Chains of 8-10 regularly.
8. Dog XXII.	"	Diplococcus.	+	+	Lower third.	—	—		Slight.	—	—	Invisible.	Same organism recovered from peritonitis.
9. Dog XXIII.	"	Sta hylococcus.	+	Slight.	Slight.	—	—	—	Slight.	—	—	Invisible.	
10. Dog XXVII.	"	Streptococcus.	+	+	Complete.	+	—	—	Slight.	—	+6 dys	Invisible.	
11. Dog XXVII.	"	Staphy. albus.	+	Slight.	+	—	—	—	Considerable,	—	—	Dry white.	
12. Dog XXVIII.	"	Diplococcus.	+	Slight.	Lower half.	Gelatinous.	—	—	Slight.	—	—	Spread'g.	
13. Dog XXXII.	"	Streptococcus.	+	+	Lower half.	—	—	—	Slight p. p.	—	—	Invisible.	Peculiar morphology. Long chains
14. Dog XXXII.	"	Streptococcus.	+	Slight.	Lower 4-fifths.	—	—	—	Slight.	—	—	Invisible.	

There is a conspicuous absence in surgical literature of any corresponding notes upon the microbic contents of the intestine, the lumen of which has been exposed for operative purposes. In the elaborate monograph on peritonitis by Tavel and Lanz it is noted that one case of pyloric resection in Professor Kocher's clinic was found to have a sterile duodenum; and one observation upon the peritoneal flora of a perforating duodenal ulcer showed streptococci and a yeast, two organisms commonly present in the duodenum and rarely found, alone at all events, as the result of a perforating ulcer farther down in the canal.[1]

It does not come within the scope of this paper, however, to discuss the relative prognoses in lesions resultant to pathological perforations, nor indeed to consider pathological conditions of the bowel in any way other than to show that the flora of these states, as well as of normal ones, may be diminished or altered by suitable precautions preliminary to operation. It is undoubtedly due to the fact that the customary preparation for ether with its limited diet leaves in the majority of cases the upper part of the canal comparatively free from bacteria, that operations in this part of the canal carry with them a much more favorable prognosis than others which, while in themselves no more severe, deal with lower portions of the intestine, where infected sutures, fistulæ and peritoneal complications are more common sequelæ.

Upon several occasions it will be seen that under ordinary methods of dietary preparations for anæsthesia, as in Case I, the intestinal lumen with a normal muscosa has been found at operation free from bacteria. Again, by precautionary feeding, it has been found possible to bring about this condition with apparent certainty. In other cases, many of them representing states of chronic gastritis from ulcer, carcinoma, dilatations, etc., with a percentage of HCl varying from complete absence to a degree of hyperacidity, we have been occasionally able to render the stomach and upper bowel completely free from those bacteria whose growth had been fostered by the pathological process. The procedure which

[1] It has been our experience to find that the peritonitides in human beings of high intestinal origin are almost invariably streptococcal in character, whereas after low perforations the prevalence of B. coli in the exudate is aften sufficient to obscure the presence of any other accompanying organisms.

we have employed is simple and mainly consists in an attempt to render amicrobic all ingesta. The mouth is rinsed with an antiseptic solution and the teeth are carefully brushed at intervals of a few hours and with especial care before and after feeding. The stomach, if any chronic catarrh exists and micro-organisms in number are found present after a test meal, is washed out carefully morning and evening. Food is taken in small amounts and at comparatively frequent intervals, from clean or, preferably, sterile vessels and consists of boiled water, sterilized milk, beef-tea, albumen-water and similar liquids. Patients with chronic gastritis have been seen to gain in weight under this régime. Preliminary to the operation for from six to ten hours nothing is given by the mouth, rectal feeding being instituted if necessary.

In our first case, operated upon February 14, 1898, after the usual dietary precautions for anæsthesia, the duodenum was unexpectedly found to be free from bacteria on coverslips and in cultures. A similar condition is illustrated in Case II.

Case. I. Surgical No. 7411. *Resection of primary carcinoma of duodenal papilla. Cultures from duodenum and gall-bladder.*

After the usual preparation for ether with abstinence from solid food for eighteen hours and a fast of six hours, an exploratory laparotomy was made by Prof. Halsted, disclosing a distended gall-bladder and a small carcinoma of the duodenal papilla which had caused a complete biliary obstruction. The tumor was resected with portions of the duodenum and of the biliary and pancreatic ducts. The bowel was closed with transplantation of the amputated ducts into the line of suture. Recovery was uneventful. Cultures and coverslips from the gall-bladder, common duct and duodenum, were negative for micro-organisms.

This case was most exceptional from a surgical standpoint, and instructive from a bacteriological one. Obstruction of the common duct by a stone is almost invariably associated with periodical infections of the biliary apparatus of greater or less severity which presumably occasion the subsequent contraction of the gall-bladder in these cases. Similarly, experimental ligation of the common duct, as has been shown by Netter (Le Progrès Médicale, 1886) and others, is followed by infection and cholangitis. Here there existed a complete obstruction with dilatation of the gall-bladder unassociated with biliary infection. The case, furthermore, is of importance in that it shows that the duodenum may be found sterile under conditions which absolutely eliminate the possibility that any antiseptic property of the bile may have been the causative agent.

Case II. Surgical No. 9222. *Gall-stone impacted in ampulla of Vater. Cultures from biliary passages and duodenum.*

For the removal of the " ball valve " gall-stone in this case it was necessary to incise the duodenum over the duct. Only the usual dietary precautions preliminary to ether had been taken. The duodenum was empty and cultures from its mucous surface proved microscopically and culturally negative. Cultures from the common duct, gall-bladder and centre of the stone were also sterile, though only a month's interval had elapsed since the last attack of intermittent fever of biliary origin. It has been our invariable rule to make at the time of operation a microscopical examination of the contents of opened ducts and intestine in such cases as this, since negative findings corresponding to the above may greatly alter the operator's attitude toward the peritoneal toilet before closure.

The following case was one of the early ones in which bacteriological examinations were made and was operated upon without the dietary precautions which subsequently were instituted. It illustrates that in some pathological states, at all events, the usual dietary preparation may not affect the organisms present in the canal and that these may be the cause of an ensuing peritonitis.

Case III. Surgical No. 7817. *Excision of cicatrizing ulcer of pylorus. Cultures from stomach and duodenum.*

The patient had a greatly dilated stomach and had had gastric hemorrhages; a pyloric tumor could be palpated. After an Ewald test breakfast, 500 cc. of bad-smelling material was recovered containing free HCl in 10 cc. sufficient to neutralize 3.5 cc. of $\frac{N}{10}$ NaOH solution. A great variety of bacteria were also present. A pylorectomy was performed by Dr. Halsted after Billroth's method.

Bacteriological study of intestine at operation.—Microscopical examination of the stomach contents showed an abundant and most polymorphic flora; many spirilla faintly staining and a great variety of bacilli which decolorized by Gram; varieties of cocci in groups, pairs and short chains, as well as some short bacilli, which did not decolorize. In the duodenal contents comparatively few bacteria were seen: yeast granules, a few cocci, some in pairs, and an occasional short strepto-bacillus. None apparently decolorized by Gram's stain. In agar appeared a few colonies of a liquefying coccus (Staphylococcus albus) and an orange-colored yeast.

The patient died on the second day, not having rallied from the operation. At autopsy the suture was found intact. No marked evidence of peritonitis was present, but coverslips from the serosa in the region of the operation showed a great number of bacteria, chiefly staphylococci and bacilli of the colon type. On culture were isolated a great number of colonies of Staphylococcus albus and an actively motile non-liquefying bacillus with colon morphology, but which produced no gas, did not coagulate milk and formed abundant indol. The same bacteria also were isolated from spleen and kidneys.

That the gastric and duodenal flora may be so far diminished by dietary precautions even in pathological states as to greatly lessen the possibility of an ensuing peritonitis is shown by the following four cases, which may be contrasted with the preceding one.

Case IV. Surgical No. 8703. *Pyloroplasty for stenosis. Cultures from stomach and duodenum.*

The patient, a young woman, aged 28, was operated upon by Prof. Halsted, March 11, 1899, for gastric symptoms, which were found to have been occasioned by a pyloric stenosis. Considerable dilatation of the stomach was present, and a test breakfast showed a total acidity of 6 with 4.4 of free hydrochloric acid. On microscopical examination were found numerous yeast cells, diplococci and pleomorphic bacilli. Several subsequent observations gave practically the same results with the occasional addition of staphylococcus clumps. Cultures, however, taken from the gastric contents recovered after these test meals, expressed through a stomach-tube, proved sterile in agar on three occasions.

At the time of operation, which was some hours after taking nourishment, stained preparations were negative for bacteria, and cultures remained sterile except for one colony of a skin coccus (Staphylococcus albus), probably a contamination.

Preliminary bacteriological examinations in this case, though it was one of chronic gastritis, had shown the high percentage of HCl present and the consequent condition of microbic sterility even during the early digestion (one hour after the test breakfast) of an unsterilized though simple meal. No especial dietary precautions were taken before operation except the usual six hours' abstinence from food. Convalescence was without abdominal symptoms.

Case V. Surgical No. 8492. *Dilatation of stomach from pyloric stenosis. Cultures from stomach and duodenum after precautionary feeding.*

A stricture of the pylorus of uncertain origin had existed in this case for many months with resultant dilatation of the stomach and chronic gastritis. A test breakfast ordinarily gave a return of 100 to 200 cc. of material after one hour with an excess of free HCl. The stomach was washed out regularly night and morning and the patient was put upon amicrobic diet for five days before the operation. There was a gain in weight of one pound a day under this régime. At the end of this period a plastic operation on the pylorus was made by Dr. Halsted and stomach and duodenum were opened. Cultures from both situations were sterile.

Case VI. Surgical No. 8226. *Partial excision of stomach and pylorus for carcinoma.*

In this case, Henry W., aged 56, no preliminary bacteriological examination had been made of the gastric contents. There was complete absence of HCl on several examinations and presumably a fairly abundant gastric flora. The stomach was thoroughly washed out on several occasions before the operation and rectal feeding instituted. The tumor, including a large portion of the stomach and pylorus, was excised by Dr. Finney. Cultures and coverslips were taken from the duodenum alone and proved sterile. The patient died several days later, consequent to an ether pneumonia. At the autopsy the suture was found intact, free from surrounding adhesions, and cultures from the neighboring serosa were negative.

Case VII. Surgical No. 8835. *Gastro-enterostomy for carcinoma of stomach. Dietary precautions taken. Cultures from stomach and jejunum.*

The patient presented an inoperable carcinoma of the stomach. Examinations of stomach contents after Ewald test breakfasts had shown a complete absence of HCl, and on microscopic examination a large number of pleomorphic bacteria. Many bacilli had the morphological characteristics of the Oppler-Boas variety. Stomach washings and precautionary diet were instituted, and at the operation, performed by Dr. Finney, cultures and coverslips from the jejunum were negative. On examination of the stomach contents the microscope showed a few bacilli, which decolorized by Gram, and an occasional coccus. Only four cultures grew out on an aërobic plate, two of them yeasts; the others were unidentified.

The following case is given to illustrate the fact that the presence of streptococci among the microbic varieties in the stomach render these precautions before operation the more necessary.

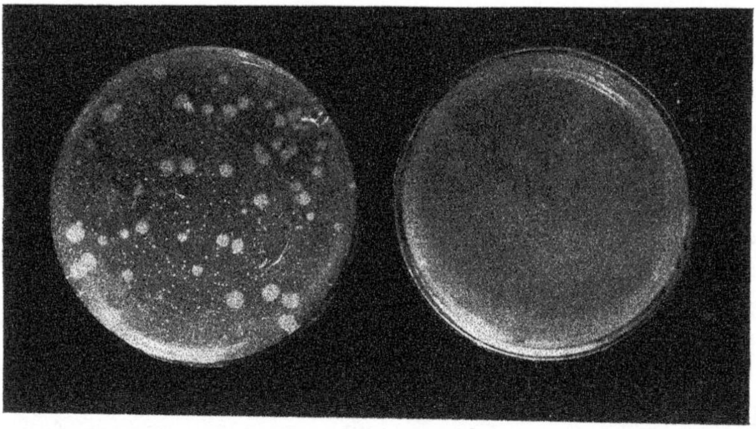

FIG. 1.—Case VIII. Surg. No. 8623. Agar plates from stomach contents. I. February 3, 1899. Before dietary precautions. The visible colonies are bacillary ones. The myriads of fine streptococcus colonies in the depth are unfortunately obscured by the mesh of the half tone screen. II. February 8, 1899. Sterile plate after five days of precautionary feeding.

Case VIII. Surgical No. 8623. *Duodenal stenosis following cholelithiasis, with dilatation of the stomach and submucous distension ulcer. Cultures from stomach and distension pouch.*

This case was one of great interest from a bacteriological and surgical standpoint. The patient, a man aged 36, had for some years suffered from symptoms of gastric dilatation. The inflated stomach reached some distance below the umbilicus and measured 31 cm. in its long diameter. A large amount of material (400 to 500 cc.) could be recovered after test breakfasts (Ewald) which might or might not show free HCl. Microscopical examination of this fluid showed a great number of bacteria, polymorphous bacilli, many with Oppler-Boas morphology, and a great number of diplo- and streptococci. Cultures were upon several occasions taken from this material into agar as it was expressed through a sterile stomach-tube and immediately plated. On the first occasion (cf. Fig. 1), Feb. 3, 1899, there developed a great number of colonies chiefly of two varieties: several hundred colonies in depth and on the surface of a motile bacillus with the morphology of B. coli, while in the depth of the media also were a multitude of fine colonies proving to be streptococci. For a period of five days preliminary to the operation the dietary precautions heretofore described were instituted. The number of bacteria diminished rapidly from the stomach under lavage and sterile feeding, and on the day before the laparotomy but few bacteria and no streptococci were found in the recovered material of the test meal and the plate (cf. Fig. 1), Feb. 8, 1899, remained sterile.

At the operation Dr. Halsted found a dense mass of adhesions about the region of the gall-bladder, pylorus and duodenum, which had held up the latter and caused the stenosis. In separating these adhesions to free the duodenum and to remove the gall-stones, which were found to be the occasion of the trouble, a small opening was made into what was supposed to be the lumen of the adherent stomach, since there escaped from it a considerable amount of white mucoid material. This opening was immediately closed. Cover-slip preparations and cultures from this material contained a great number of streptococcus chains. The operation was satisfactorily concluded, after liberating the adherent duodenum and removing the gall-stones. The patient died in 48 hours from a general streptococcus peritonitis and septicæmia. It was found at autopsy, by Dr. MacCallum, that the presumable opening into the lumen of the stomach, which was naturally at the time of operation supposed to be practically amicrobic, had in reality led into a large submucous distension ulcer near the pylorus which was full of streptococci; this diverticulum had escaped the cleansing process which the rest of the viscus had undergone.

The very fact of an ensuing peritonitis in this case, through the accidental opening of an anomalous and rare diverticulum containing pathogenic bacteria which had escaped our precautionary measures directed towards the stomach, and which, after all, did not need to be opened, only emphasizes by its irony the principles involved in our communication.

The following cases are given to show that the condition of amicrobism may extend to the upper portion of the jejunum.

Case IX. Surgical No. 9083. *Pylorectomy and gastrojejunostomy for carcinoma. Cultures from stomach and jejunum.*

At the operation in this case an adenocarcinoma of the posterior wall of the stomach and pylorus was found. There was but slight chronic gastritis, and free hydrochloric acid was present on the examination of a test meal. Only the usual dietary preparations for anæsthesia were taken, and yet at operation from the stomach contents very few organisms were cultivated. Cultures showed colonies of yeast and an unidentified bacillus. From the jejunal contents no organisms were found with the microscope. One agar plate remained sterile: the other gave several colonies of the same bacillus which was found in the stomach. It decolorized by Gram and did not coagulate milk. No cocci whatever could be demonstrated.

Case X. Surgical No. 9087. *Perforating bullet wound of abdomen. Lesions in jejunum and transverse colon. Cultures from jejunal contents.*

The patient had been shot seven hours before his admission and laparotomy. Some time had elapsed since the taking of food, but nevertheless the lower lacteals were injected and showed some activity in digestion in the lower intestine. A double perforation was present in the jejunum a short distance below the duodenum, and two similar lesions were found in the transverse colon. From the latter site apparently no extravasation of contents had taken place. The material which appeared at the jejunal openings, and which had soiled the neighboring serosa, contained a great number of polymorphonuclear leucocytes, but on microscopical examination was apparently free from micro-organisms. Cultures taken from it remained sterile. Recovery was uneventful.

Our introductory remarks suffice to explain the absence of serious peritoneal complications in such cases of high perforation occurring at the end of digestion. A lesson may be drawn from the lesions in the colon, namely, that perforations of the large bowel in conditions of health are often unassociated with extravasation on account of the semi-solid character of the contents and probably not infrequently may be recovered from, without operative intervention, through the agency of protecting omental adhesions.

Case XI. Surgical No. 9476. *Exploratory laparotomy for carcinoma of the stomach. Jejunostomy. Cultures from jejunum after sterile feeding.*

The patient was operated upon when in an extreme condition, since he was unable to retain any food given by the mouth. Preliminary stomach-washings did not seem to materially affect the gastric flora. There was complete absence of free HCl. An operation with the intention of performing a gastro-enterostomy

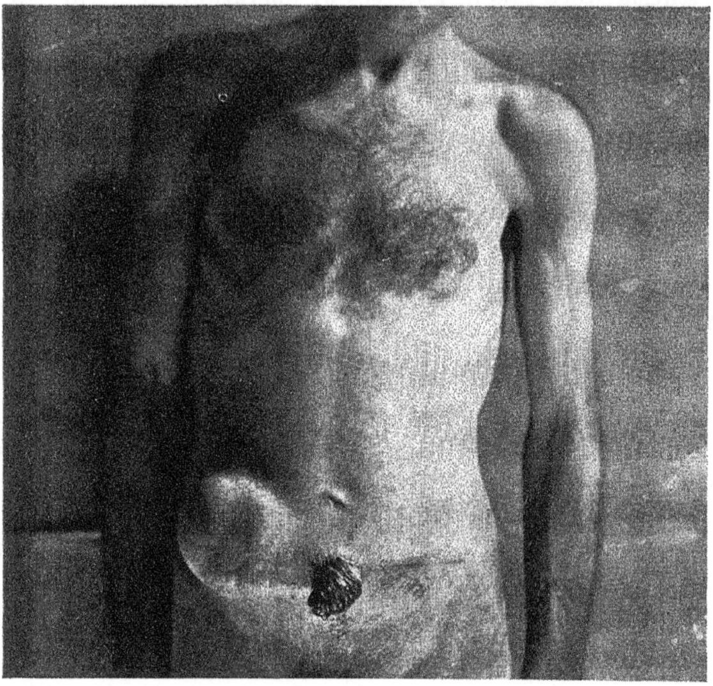

FIG. 2.—Case XII. Surg. No. 8025. Showing situation of fistula and prolapse of mucous membrane during a period of fasting; also large ventral hernia.

was undertaken. The stomach was found contracted and too extensively involved to permit of an anastomosis. The first coil of jejunum was brought out above the transverse colon and a jejunostomy for feeding purposes was established by the method of Witzel, as ordinarily employed in the stomach. The jejunum was empty at the time of opening and a scraping of its surface gave no bacteria in culture. An almost complete obstruction must have existed at the pylorus. The small intestine below was empty and apparently free from micro-organisms.

The following cases of jejunal fistulæ demonstrate the fact that a state of amicrobism may be brought about which extends for some distance below the duodenum.

Case XII. Surgical No. 8025. *High almost complete jejunal fistula. Sterilized feeding preliminary to intestinal resection. Cultures from both limbs of fistula.*

This case presented many features of unusual interest, some clinical notes concerning which have been already briefly reported

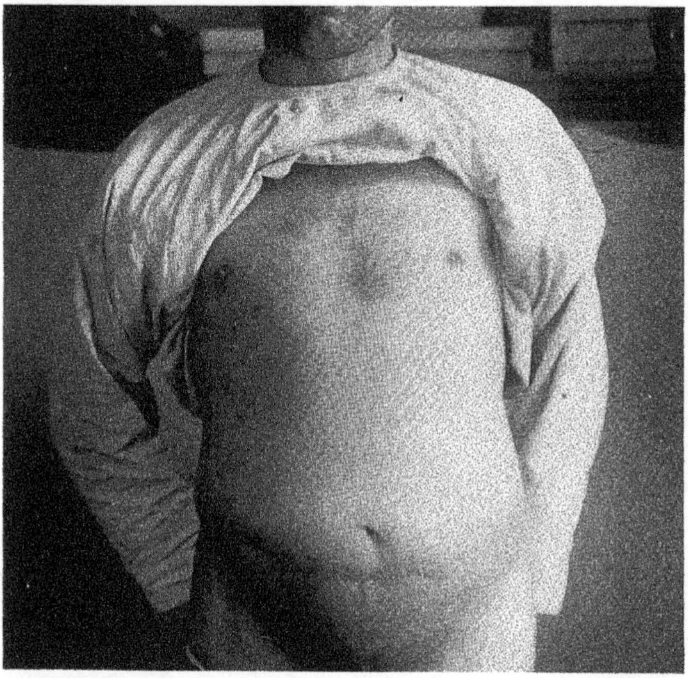

FIG. 3.—Case XII. Condition two months after operation, with gain in weight of 88½ pounds.

(Johns Hopkins Hospital Bulletin, July, 1899). A fistula, situated about 12 inches below the duodenum, through which almost the entire products of digestion escaped, had existed for years as the result of an incised wound across the abdomen (cf. Fig. 2). Liquid food given by the mouth could be recovered in a very short time after ingestion; a glass of milk, for example, on one occasion given on an empty stomach began to appear, acid in reaction and finely coagulated, at the fistula in one minute and was entirely recovered in four minutes. Cultures taken from the discharging products of the fistula during active digestion showed a diversity of organisms. Dr. Clopton on one occasion isolated the following organisms: B. coli communis, the predominating form, B. lactis aërogenes, B. pyocyaneus, B. proteus, two unidentified bacilli and

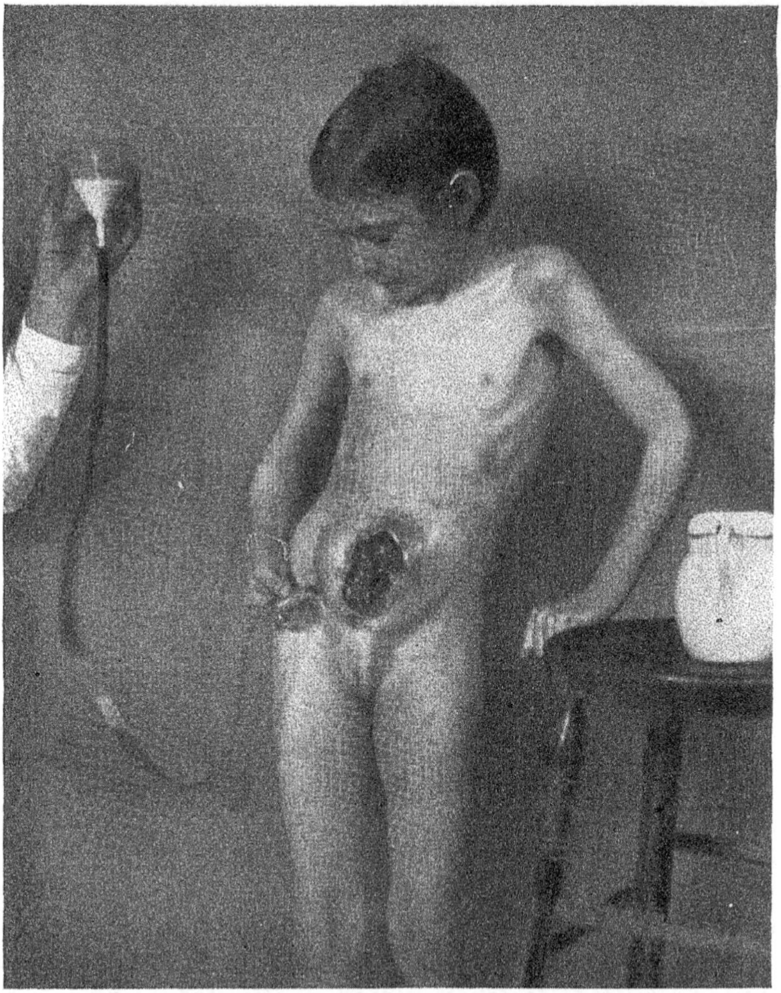

FIG. 4.—Case XIII. Showing jejunal fistula with prolapse of mucous membrane most marked in the distal limb; also method of feeding at lower fistula established for that purpose.

some varieties of yeasts. From over-feeding, a chronic catarrhal condition of the stomach was present, and the percentage of HCl in the gastric juice was found to be most variable. As a consequence, the antiseptic action of gastric digestion could not be depended upon to materially affect introduced bacteria. It nevertheless was found that, by instituting a régime of sterilized feeding,

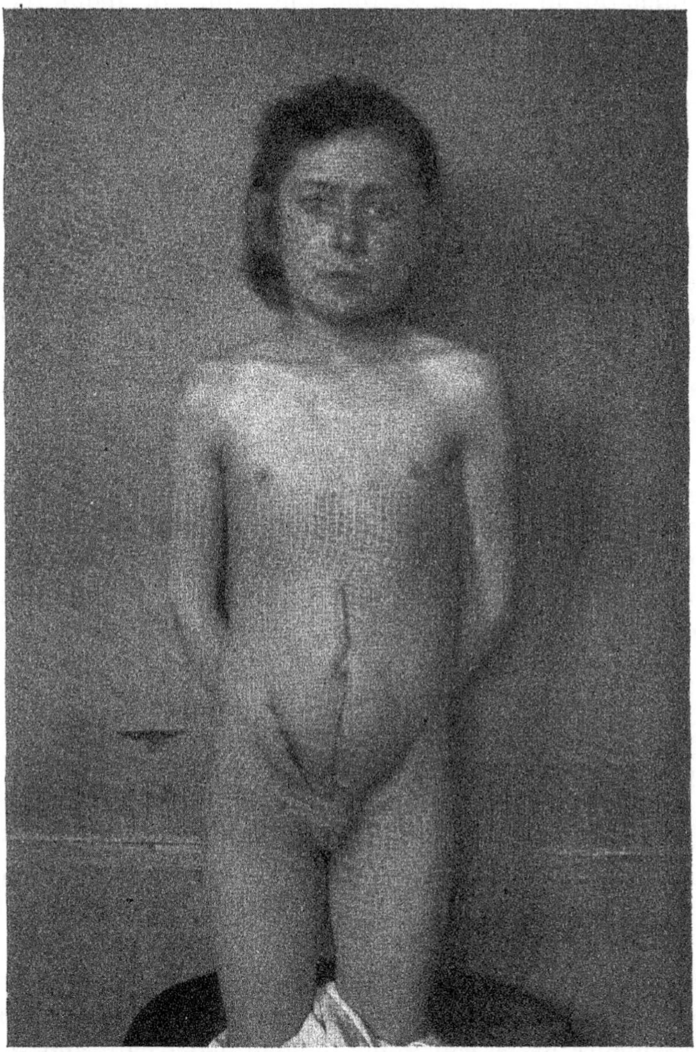

FIG. 5.—Case XIII. After sixth laparotomy which had been performed for the relief of acute appendicitis and its complications.

the number and variety of the organisms recoverable at the fistula could be materially diminished. On resumption of his usual diet the pleomorphic and abundant flora would return. On various occasions milk, inoculated with chromogenic organisms, as B. prodigiosus,[1] B. zanthemis and Staphylococcus pyogenes aureus, was given and the organisms could be recovered during the period of active discharge of the milk from the fistula in about the same number as in the medium introduced, and only toward the last period of escape did the number of colonies diminish and the original organisms reassert themselves. Possibly owing to the exposure of the mucous membrane at the site of the fistula and the consequent catarrhal condition, the surface could never be rendered amicrobic and some bacteria could always be recovered. Nevertheless, after a period of sterilized diet even on this surface they were greatly reduced in number, and at the time of operation and resection of the bowel at an opening six inches above the fistula, microscopical examination was negative and cultures from the mucous membrane remained sterile. The abdomen was closed without drainage (cf. Fig. 3).

Case XIII. Surgical No. 8513. *Complete high jejunal fistula. Dietary precautions preliminary to resection of the bowel. Cultures from both limbs of fistula.*

A child, aged 10, while convalescing from an extensive peritonitis, due to a perforated appendix, was seized with symptoms of acute intestinal obstruction. At the time of operation, three days later, a mass of small intestine was found with one distended coil of jejunum leading to it and another, collapsed, leading away from it. In the vain attempt to disentangle the adherent loops which were densely matted together, several holes were torn into the bowel. The prostrated condition of the patient forbade a prolonged operation, and the whole mass, consisting of about two feet of jejunum, was excised and the free ends of the bowel were left in the wound. Microscopical examination of the contents of the bowel, which had become backed up by obstruction, showed, as is usual in such cases, a great number of micro-organisms. From a dilution of this material into an agar plate there developed many hundred colonies of B. coli, some unidentified bacilli and streptococci. Unfortunately the proximal limb of the fistula, as was subsequently found, was situated so high in the jejunum that, as in the previous case, all nourishment was lost soon after its entry into the

[1] Macfayden (loc. cit.) has shown that B. prodigiosus is one of the most susceptible of organisms to the action of the gastric juice.

stomach. Closure of the fistula was postponed for some months, during which it was hoped many of the adhesions would become absorbed. In the interim the patient lived in the condition shown in the photograph (Fig. 4), spending her nights in a constant bath, since it was necessary to keep her under water many hours out of the twenty-four in order to control the severe dermatitis which the discharge produced. She was nourished, meanwhile, by nutritive enemata and by feeding through a fistula, which was established for this purpose at the site of the original appendix incision. A mechanical twist of the bowel unfortunately prevented the insertion of a tube into the distal limb of the jejunal fistula. The portion of small intestine, therefore, between these two points remained empty for some months.

Observations were made from time to time upon the physical and bacteriological characteristics under different dietary conditions of the material which passed through the stomach and was collected at the fistula. The bacteriological notes were made by Dr. Clopton. A variety of micro-organisms, most of which stained by Gram, always including yeasts and a very long streptococcus form, were invariably found in the acid and bile-stained material which came in jets from the fistula after taking food. The latter organisms had apparently become established at the time of the ileus and proved difficult to eliminate. Plates taken under ordinary conditions showed a multitude of colonies. A solid diet was discharged so slowly that apparently it afforded a medium in which the retained bacteria could multiply. Their number, however, diminished toward the end of digestion. On one occasion, an hour after a meal, 600 colonies of streptococci, B. coli and other unidentified bacteria were recovered from a single loop full of material; in three hours but 300 colonies developed in the same amount of material. On a liquid and sterilized diet the number dropped off more quickly. Preliminary to the operation for some days a sterilized milk diet was given. On the first day, three hours after feeding, 200 colonies, chiefly streptococcus, with colon and an unidentified streptobacillus were recovered (cf. Fig. 6). After five days, under the same conditions, there developed on the plate only nine colonies, three large surface ones of yeast and colon, and six in the depth of streptococci, yeast and colon (Fig. 7). At the time of operation, three days later, all nourishment having been discontinued by the mouth for twelve hours, both proximal and distal loops of the bowel leading to the fistula, at a distance of about six inches from it, were found to be free from micro-organisms (Fig. 8). The fistula was excised, a lateral entero-anastomosis made, and the abdominal wall closed without drainage. Recovery was uneventful (cf. Fig. 5).

The observation upon the amicrobic state of the distal loop of the fistula at a short distance from its exposed end was unexpected.

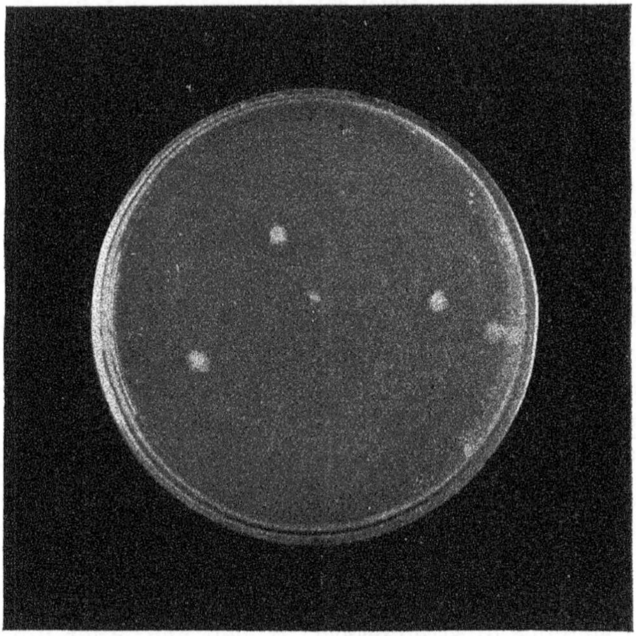

Fig. 6.—Case XIII. Agar plate inoculated from discharge at fistula three hours after first sterile feeding preliminary to operation. Two hundred colonies, chiefly of streptococci are distributed about the margin.

It nevertheless tends to confirm the results which had been obtained under other conditions in which complete emptiness of the canal could be brought about, namely, that such a state is associated with a gradual elimination of bacteria. Even farther down in the canal the same result may be observed. In a case of low jejunal fistula, established for the relief of a strangulated hernia, it was found at the time of resection and suture some weeks later, that the distal bowel at the site of anastomosis, six or eight inches from the fistula, failed to show any bacteria on coverslip or culture (cf. Report of this case in full with plates in the Annals of Surgery, January, 1900, p. 18, Case XXII).

In contrast to the case which introduces this paper and to these fistula cases, in which the intestinal contents had been rendered sterile or were found free from micro-organisms and in an empty state, the following case of jejunal rupture may be cited, since it illustrates the rapidly fatal form of peritonitis which may follow

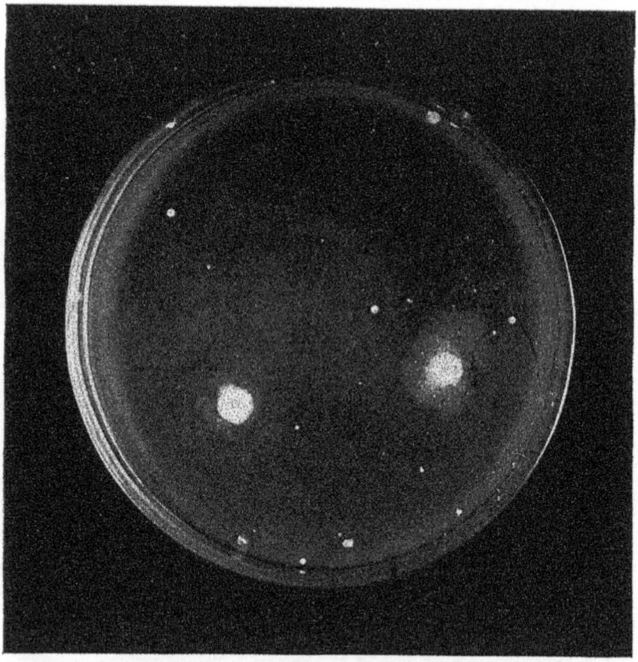

FIG. 7.—Case XIII. Plate inoculated three hours after feeding. Sterilization of ingesta for preceding five days. Nine colonies. No pathogenic varieties.

upon extravasation of food products into the abdominal cavity during the period of active digestion, when many bacteria, and especially those pathogenic ones which escape the action of the gastric juice, are present.

Case XIV. Surgical No. 9094. *Traumatic rupture of the jejunum during active digestion. Culture at situation of lesion. General peritonitis.*

The patient was brought to the hospital a few hours after a serious fall and blow upon the abdomen, which had occurred soon after taking a hearty meal. He was in a condition of collapse, complaining of abdominal pain, and a laparotomy under cocain was performed, disclosing a tear in the jejunum a foot below the duodenum. Partially digested food was free in the abdominal cavity, and microscopical examination of the peritoneal contents near the lesion gave the appearance of a pure streptococcus culture. Thorough irrigation and cleansing of the peritoneum failed to influence the acute toxæmia resultant to the intensity of the infection. The patient died within twenty-four hours of a general streptococcus infection.

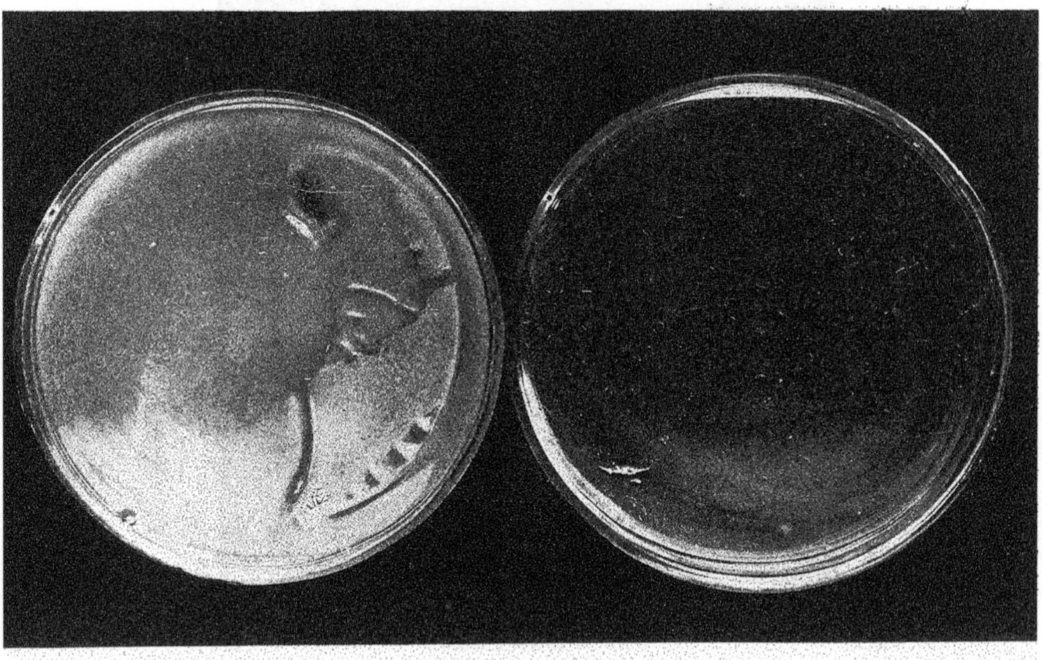

FIG. 8.—Case XIII. Sterile plates from proximal and distal bowel 18 cm. from fistula, showing condition of amicrobism at time of operation and resection.

The results of our study in its surgical relation may briefly be summarized as follows:

In the upper portion of the intestinal tract the bacterial flora is more scanty than in the lower portion.

No definite varieties of micro-organisms seem to be constant elements of this flora, which is apparently dependent upon the bacterial features of the ingesta for its characteristics.

At the terminal stages of digestion, and especially after a fast, it is difficult to recover micro-organisms from the mucous membrane of the stomach, duodenum, and even of the jejunum as far down as complete emptying of the canal has occurred.

It is of importance, therefore, by sterilization to rid the food of micro-organisms, especially of such forms as streptococci, preliminary to operative procedures; and also to insure a condition of emptiness of the upper part of the digestive tract.

As peritonitis following intestinal wounds, operative or accidental, is dependent for its characteristics upon the bacterial flora of the canal at the site of lesion, the prognosis of such conditions will be favorable proportionately with the scarcity and innocuousness of the micro-organisms which are present.

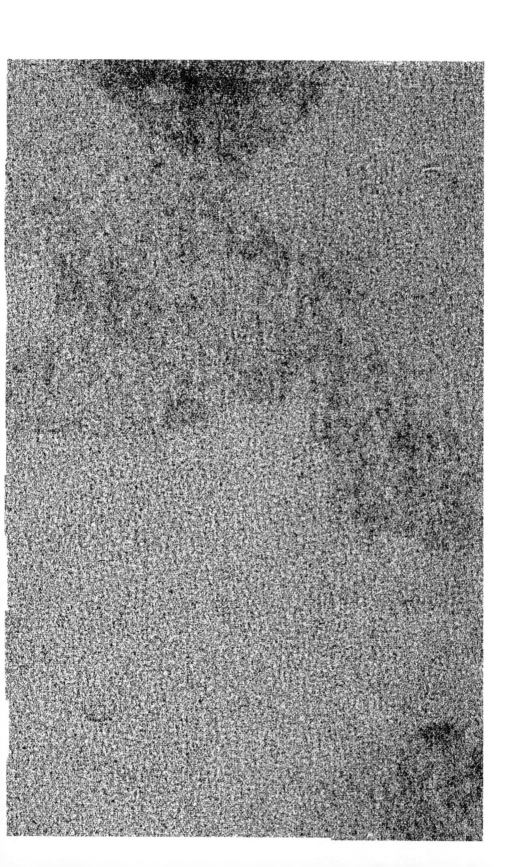

Lightning Source UK Ltd.
Milton Keynes UK
UKHW020628060119
334855UK00006B/287/P

9 780331 140286